CANINE KITCHEN CAPERS:

A Humorous Look at Preparing Food for Dogs (& Spouses)

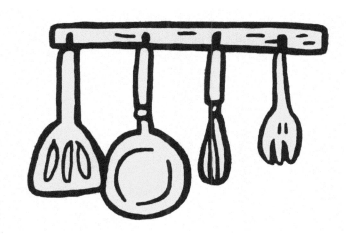

By Judy Morgan DVM and Hue Grant

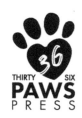

www.drjudymorgan.com

Copyright ©2016 Judy Morgan DVM and Hue Grant

Published in the United States of America

ISBN: 978-0-9972501-0-7

TABLE OF CONTENTS

INTRODUCTION

Anyone who knows me or follows my blogs knows that I often criticize the processed food industries for the horrible ingredients used in human and pet foods. High salt, sugar, and fat in processed food products are killing us all. Food waste products, 4D meats (disabled, dead, decayed, and diseased carcasses), sugars, dyes, carcinogenic preservatives, and inedible fillers are legally used routinely to make pet food.

So why do we continue to eat these products and feed them to our pets? Two words: convenience and advertising. The advertising gurus know how to put a good spin on the worst products imaginable. "Made with real beef" could mean as little as 3% of the product is actually beef. "Real beef flavor" means there is no beef, just a chemical additive to give the flavor of beef. Because consumers don't know the definitions of the words used in advertising, they are misled into thinking something is better than it really is.

My response to this dilemma: I refuse to buy processed foods from big pet food companies. For our dogs, we are left with feeding raw or home cooked foods. Puploaf is one of our favorite things to make and it's one of their favorite things to eat. Puploaf became famous and is now being made around the world.

Because many people have never cooked for their dogs, the first attempts can have comical results. Some people don't cook for themselves, some are great chefs, and some just seem to invite comedy.

I have been fortunate enough to get to laugh with my new friends undertaking this adventure. I thought it was only fair to share their exploits with the world. I hope you enjoy these stories as much as I do.

I have provided recipes for your dogs, recipes for you, and some recipes to share. Don't worry if you have a kitchen disaster. Just send me the story and maybe you can be featured in the next book!

-Judy Morgan DVM, CVA, CVCP, CVFT

I've always considered myself a foodie. Even before the Food Network made its debut, I was enamored with cooking shows on PBS, such as Jeff Smith on The Frugal Gourmet, Martin Yan on Yan Can Cook, Graham Kerr on The Galloping Gourmet, and my all-time favorite, Justin Wilson on Louisiana Cookin'. Heck, my first Boy Scout merit badge was in cooking.

I've also always considered myself an animal lover; unfortunately, though, my love of fine eating did not make its way into my dogs' bowls. Sure, they ate the veterinarian-recommended kibbles and the brands most touted by the Madison Avenue agencies in television commercials, but that was as deep as I delved into the world of pet foods. Then, I met Dr. Judy Morgan. Not only did I fall in love with her, and her beloved Cavalier King Charles Spaniels; I also became a huge fan of her pet nutrition philosophy. Before long, my treasured cooking pans became vessels for stews, puppins, and puploafs. I found myself getting excited about cooking for the Spaniels and having them clamor around my feet as I ground meat, organs, and vegetables for the latest concoction that Judy had developed. I also found myself learning about super-foods and their correlation regarding the healthy well-being of our four-legged family members. So, with my food grinder handy, my crock pot at the ready, and my loaf pans lined in a row, I now know that one of my greatest missions in life is to help Dr. Judy Morgan spread the word on good nutrition for all beings, four paws at a time.

-Hue Grant

I DID IT!

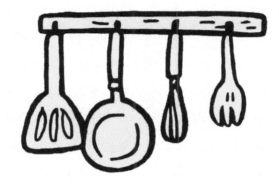

Submitted by Liz Vernon, mother to Soldier, Lexi, and Billy

I did it! Pup loaf per Dr. Judy Morgan's book. Yep, the person whose friends have been saying they want to send her to world's worst cook show. (Go ahead; I'll take the free trip).

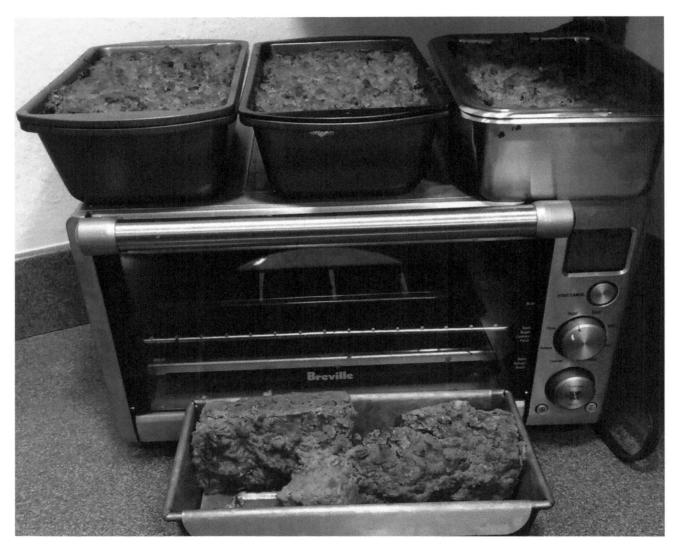

And, I did it in a toaster oven!

BURNT HUMAN, COOKED DOG

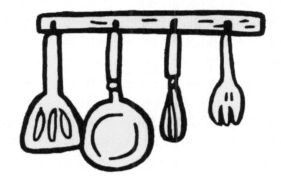

Submitted by Soldier, a Cavalier King Charles Spaniel parented by Liz Vernon

This is Soldier reporting in.

Dad was all happy cuz mom was actually making human meatloaf for him. Good; we didn't want to share ours. Dad loves meatloaf, so Mom made 4 big ones and two small ones, all for Dad. Mom burned them. Dad wants to know how she could make 16 great lookin' loafs for us and he gets charcoal-top.

Well, dimwitted Mom set the timer and took us for a walk. She knew we would get back in time. But then Mom started talking to a neighbor, and then we got to our favorite neighbor, who always gives us treats; by the time we got back, Mom had forgotten all about the loaves. Mom really shouldn't multitask; she does that all the time and crazy things happen.

Mom realized when we came in, that the timer was blaring. She really didn't need the timer; the smoky haze in the kitchen was a pretty good clue, along with the fire alarm.

So Mom hurried to get the meat loaves out and dropped one on the floor upside down. We all tried to get to it, but it had onion stuff that Mom said we couldn't have. Dad came in just as she picked it up and scraped off the black top and said dinner was done. It was still edible, Mom said. Dad ate it; he just poured catsup all over it like he does with everything Mom cooks. We think he should buy stock in Heinz. He keeps the market demand up.

What really upset Dad again, were the labels on Mom's freezer bags. Dad just hates that she labels loaves "human" or "dog" ... Mom just isn't worried about people wondering if we are cannibals or if we eat dogs. So she labeled them "burned human meatloaf" this time. Dad's still muttering that we have great looking loaves. Isn't that the way it's supposed to be?

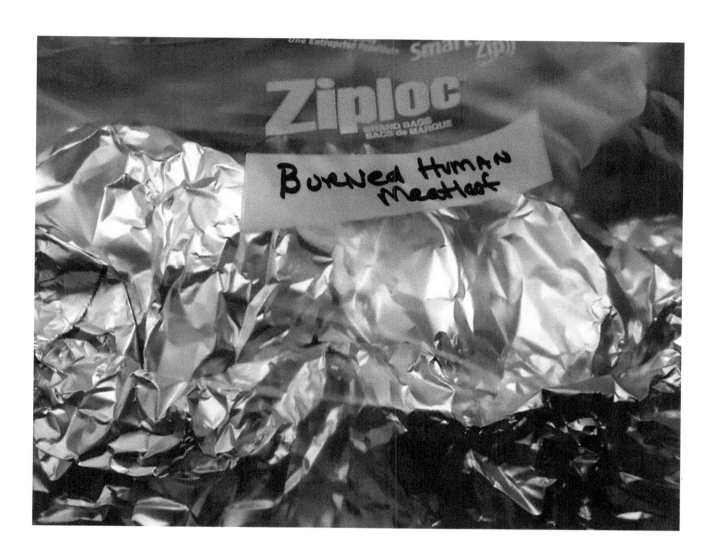

DR. MORGAN'S ORIGINAL PUPLOAF RECIPE

2 pounds lean ground meat (90% lean or higher) – beef, bison, turkey, chicken, or whatever meat you choose

½ pound ground organ meat (liver, hearts, gizzards) – this will help decrease cost and there are a lot of vitamins and nutrients in the organs that are not found in muscle meat

3 to 4 eggs to bind the ingredients

1 cup Honest Kitchen Preference, Dr. Harvey's, or similar dehydrated vegetable base rehydrated with 1 and ½ cups hot water. If preferred, you can use a cup of fresh finely chopped vegetables (no onions).

½ cup cooked barley or quinoa – not essential and can be eliminated if grain-free is your preference.

Mix all ingredients in a bowl. Place in meatloaf pan (may require two pans, depending on size) and bake at 350 degrees for 40 – 60 minutes. Should be firm, but not dry, when finished baking.

If you are not using a commercial dehydrated vegetable base with added mineral mix, you will have to add a commercial calcium/mineral supplement or 2 teaspoons of finely ground eggshells.

Most dogs will eat 2 to 3 percent of their body weight per day (about 8 – 12 ounces for a twenty pound dog).

We make big batches for 9 dogs at our house!

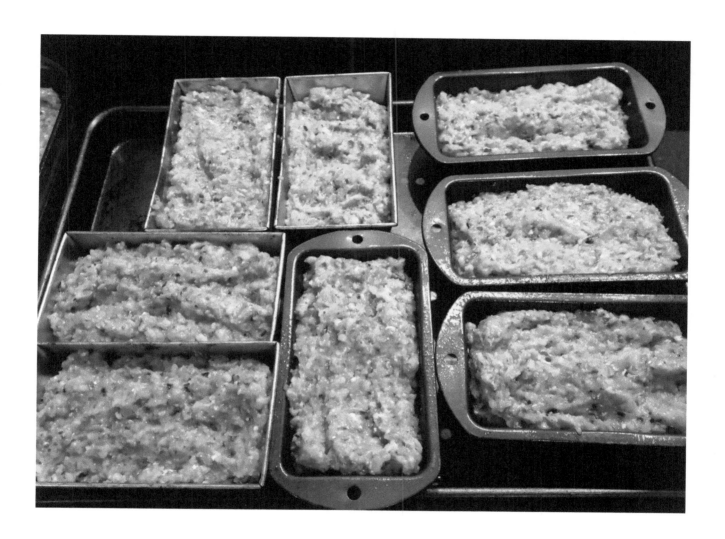

AMAZING MEATLOAF
(for Dads)

Submitted by Liz Vernon

Ground hamburger, bison, or turkey, approximately 2-4 pounds.

1 cup catsup

1 sleeve of saltines, smashed while working out aggressions

1 teaspoon A-1 Steak Sauce

1 teaspoon Worcestershire sauce

2-3 eggs, beaten

1-2 tablespoons Grey Poupon Mustard

2 teaspoons minced onions

1 envelope dry onion soup mix

(optional) ½ - 1 teaspoon minced garlic

See variation suggestions. None of these ingredients have to be exact, which is why *this* disaster cook can succeed with this.

Mix all ingredients except hamburger and crackers together. Then mix together with meat and crackers. Add variation ingredients (listed below) last. Bake 40-50 minutes, 325 degrees.

Do not forget about your meatloaf while taking dogs for a walk. If you *do* forget about it, cut off burned top and make meatloaf soup, adding water, chopped carrots, potatoes, garlic. Don't ask me about garlic cloves, I don't have a clue what to do with them. I use minced in a jar or powdered garlic.

Spinach Meatloaf Variation: Thaw out frozen spinach package. Blot out excess liquid with paper towels, add to above mix.

Another Variation: I often add a couple cups of cooked rice. I say "cooked" because I didn't cook it the first time I added rice, and unless you want a granola-type crunch to your meatloaf, cook the rice first! Duh!

Note: I always use self-draining meatloaf pans.

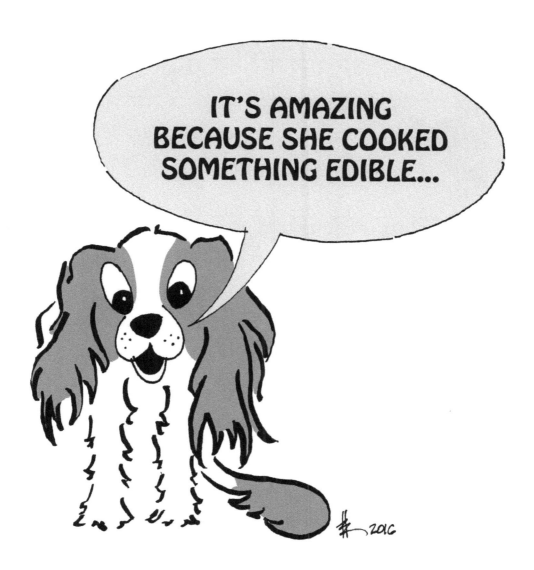

THE CASE OF
THE MISSING STEW

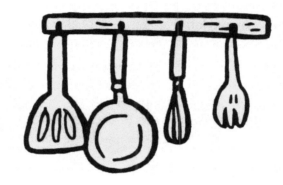

Submitted by Catherine Carmichael, mother to Oliver, Sadie, and Phoebe, 3 wonderful
Cavalier King Charles Spaniels

It was time...I knew in my heart that now was the time. After all, I had cooked home-made meals for three of my beloved Golden Retrievers when they were so sick. I had come to grips with it, but how, I asked myself, was I going to be able to do it? How was this proud vegetarian of 25 years, who had raised a daughter who was also a vegetarian, going to actually bring meat and poultry into the house after all these years? Even my husband did not get served anything that had a face. So here I was, contemplating bringing this stuff in my house, having to actually touch it and cook it, allowing the smells to permeate my walls.

It began when I starting realizing that even though I was feeding the top brands of pet food, mostly canned and not exactly cheap for three dogs, I was giving them unhealthy ingredients like carrageenan and other things I couldn't even pronounce. I didn't really know if the meat itself came from China or if the added vitamins and supplements came from somewhere other than the United States. Here I was spending a small fortune trying to keep my dogs thriving and didn't know if that was the case.

So, I purchased a nice large crock pot and lots of chicken – boneless and skinless, so that I wouldn't have to pull skin off the vile pieces. I dumped it all into my crock pot, along with lots of good veggies and barley, and cooked it all day. I went about my business, working and sewing, and soon heard crying. Running to see what was happening, I saw my Sadie sitting in the kitchen whimpering at the wonderful smells coming from that magical thing on the counter; the magical thing that was allowing me to cook this hearty, healthy meal for my three Cavaliers. All I really had to do was throw ingredients in the pot and stir it from time to time. Even the smell was more like vegetables. I was thinking this could be a great thing.

Then it came time to dish it out and let it cool for a few minutes. At that point I had three whirling dervishes and if you have ever seen a blind 10 year old dog whirl in happiness, well let's just say it makes your heart soar. It could not cool fast enough for them. And when I put their meals down, I knew I did the right thing for them. They devoured everything in their bowls, cleaning them so well that I just put them back in the cabinet. Okay, not really, I washed them first.

The next morning, I thought I would heat some of their stew in a saucepan and give it to them for break-fast. I pulled the huge bowl out of the refrigerator and was shocked at how much was gone...surely I hadn't overfed them that much last night! As I was wondering aloud, my poor, meat-starved hubby sheepishly confessed that he had tasted it the night before; and then he got himself a bowlful, which might have turned into another bowlful.

I guess I really do have a wonderful husband because he didn't complain about vegetarian cooking for the past twenty years. But after seeing how much he enjoyed the stew, I now use the crock pot all the time, making healthy yummy food for my dogs and my grateful husband.

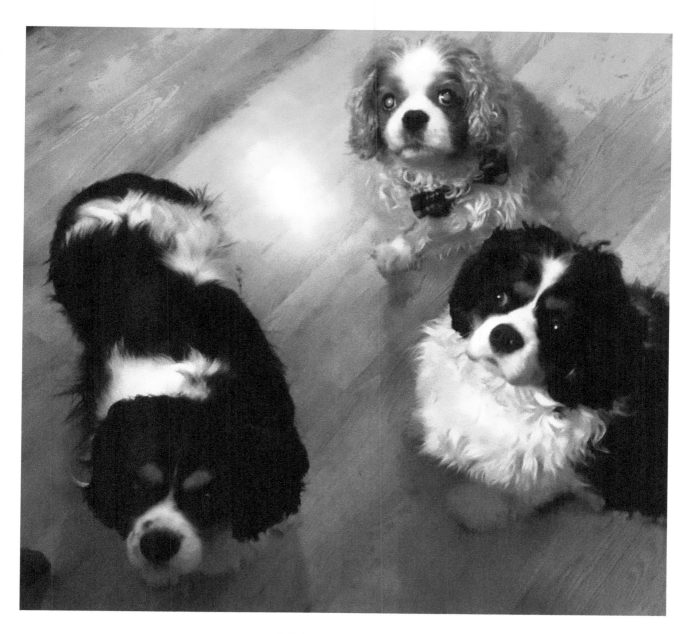

Dad did what with our stew?

CHICKEN STEW

Submitted by Judy Morgan

6 pounds of chicken - whole chicken, cut up - remove bones after cooking. By allowing the bones to cook, you get the vitamins and minerals that dissolve from the marrow. If you are squeamish, use boneless, skinless chicken. You'll also have less work to do at the end of preparation and your dogs won't have to stare at you as long, while waiting for you to finish making their meal.

2.5 pounds of chicken livers cut up. If you can't touch them, just dump them in whole.

1.25 pounds of chicken gizzards and hearts cut up. These aren't as gross as liver, but you can toss them in whole if you need to.

3 parsnips – peeled and sliced. If you don't know what a parsnip is, use carrots.

2 sweet potatoes – peeled and sliced. They are pretty similar to yams, so you could use those if so inclined.

1/3 pound of kale or spinach, chopped

5 ounces of Shiitake mushrooms, chopped

2 apples – peeled and cored. I'm partial to Fuji, but it's your choice.

Mix all ingredients in a 12 quart pot and add water to cover. Simmer for 2 to 3 hours.

Add 1 cup of steel cut oats one hour before end of cooking, unless you want a grain-free stew, in which case you should not add oats.

When finished cooking, allow to cool, remove bones and cut up chicken. Add a mineral mix at the time of feeding or use ground egg shells at the rate of 1/2 teaspoon per pound of meat. Give your dog 1/8th teaspoon of fermented cod liver oil per 10 pounds of body weight three times per week to supplement Vitamin D and omega 3's with this diet.

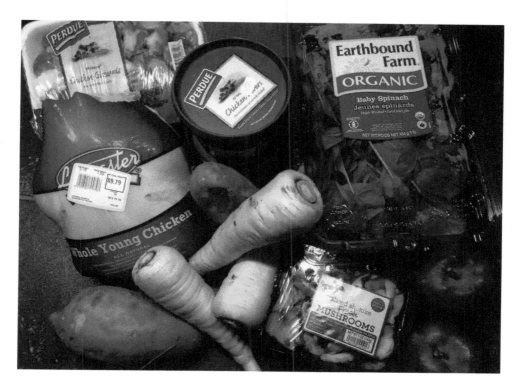

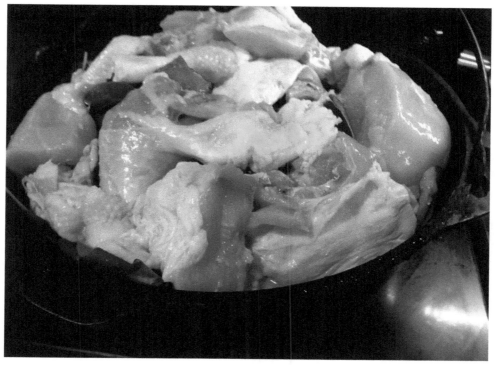

HUE STUE aka BRUNSWICK STEW
Submitted by Hue Grant

(This recipe takes a long time to make, but it's worth it! Please do not share with your dogs.)

4 pound Whole Chicken

2 pounds Pork Loin

2 pounds Beef Brisket

5 ounces Worcestershire Sauce

4 ounces Wine Vinegar

4 ounces Rice Vinegar

7 - 9 large Whole Ripe Tomatoes

1 small Red Pepper seeded

4 Vidalia Onions

10 – 12 ounces White Corn kernels (fresh or frozen)

10 – 12 ounces Lima Beans (fresh or frozen)

10 – 12 ounces Okra (fresh or frozen)

6 medium cloves Garlic minced

24 ounces Chicken Broth

24 ounces Ketchup

10 ounces Steak Sauce

¼ cup firmly packed Brown Sugar

3 large Lemons juiced

1 tablespoon Salt

1 tablespoon Pepper

1 tablespoon Hot Pepper Sauce

Smoke chicken 2.5 hours; smoke pork loin and beef brisket 6 hours. Remove chicken from bone. Chop chicken, pork, and beef.

Stir together meats and remaining ingredients in a large Dutch oven. Cook slowly on top of stove, covered, stirring every 30 minutes or so, for 8 hours. Then refrigerate for 24 hours and re-heat before serving.

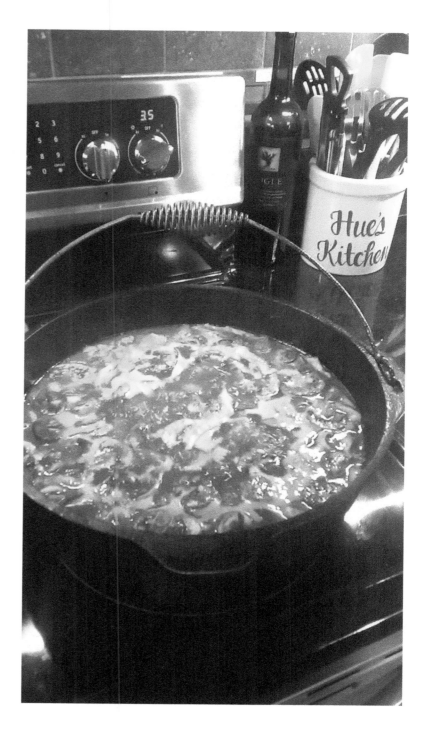

SWEATERS IN THE OVEN

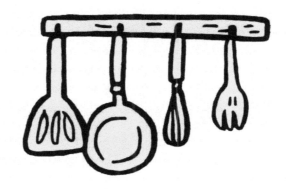

Submitted by Linda Phillips

My name is Linda Phillips and I live with a tri-colored cavalier named Valentino. I am vegan and can't stand the look or feel of meat. When Dr. Judy was giving me recipes for Valentino, just the thought of going into the butcher store freaked me out. I didn't cook for myself! I informed Dr. Morgan that my oven was the place where I stored my sweaters. After all, storage space was limited. That hole in the wall was a great place to store extra clothing. She looked at me like I had just spoken in a foreign language, but smiled and moved forward with instructions. To get started on my new venture, Dr. Judy was nice enough to give me a few ways to improve the quality of meals for my beloved pup without having to actually cook.

But with time, I decided I needed to be brave. I cleared the sweaters from the oven and headed out to buy meat. I arrived home with all the ingredients and it was time to prepare the meal. I put on three pairs of rubber kitchen gloves and two aprons to prepare the meat. There was no way I wanted any of it touching any part of my skin or clothing. The things we do for our little fur babies! Valentino stood by the oven and his little sniffer was going crazy while his puploaf was cooking. He was in doggie heaven!

When I served Valentino his first home cooked meal, he licked his bowl like never before. He looked up at me and begged for more. It was a very proud moment – I had made my pup happy!

Now, he parks himself next to the oven and patiently waits for the timer to go off, telling me his food is done. I never have to worry about overcooking because as soon as that timer dings my little guy starts barking like crazy! Needless to say, it's all worth it, for the love we have for our little ones. Thank you Dr. Judy for creating such a healthy and enjoyable meal for my little Valentino!

-"Some succeed because they are destined to... Most succeed because they are determined to." -unknown

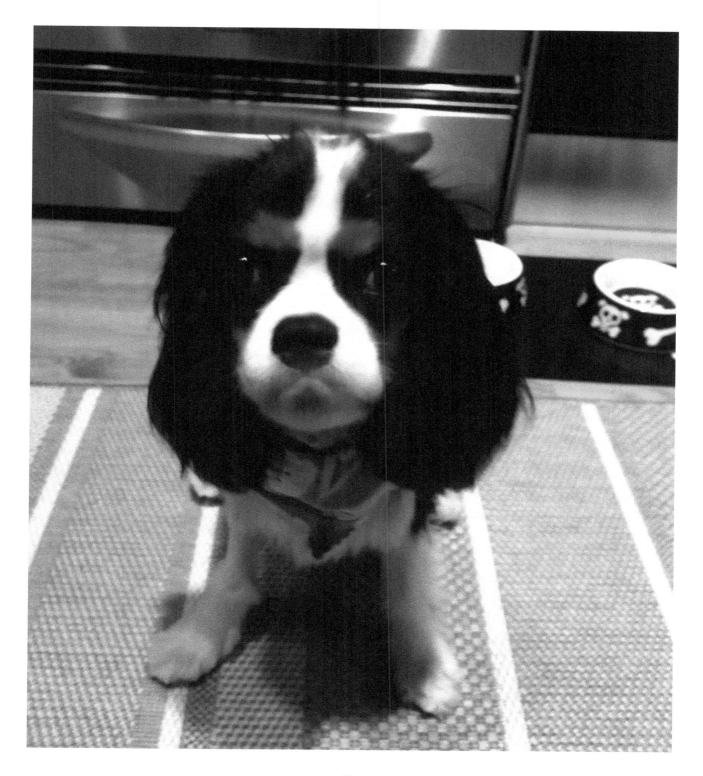

TURKEY MEATLOAF FOR TWO (SHARABLE)

Submitted by Hue Grant

Ingredients

1 cup Panko bread crumbs

1/2 cup milk

1 egg, beaten

1 stalk celery, finely chopped

1 small carrot, finely chopped

1/4 cup dried cranberries

1/2 teaspoon salt

1/4 teaspoon pepper

3 teaspoons minced fresh sage

3 teaspoons minced fresh rosemary

1-1/2 pounds lean ground turkey

1/2 cup whole-berry cranberry sauce

1/2 cup ketchup

Directions

Preheat oven to 375°. In a large bowl, combine bread crumbs and milk. Stir in egg, celery, carrot, cranberries, salt and pepper. Combine sage and rosemary; add half to the mixture. Add ground turkey and mix well. Pat into an ungreased 9x5-inch loaf pan.

Bake, uncovered, 25 minutes; drain if necessary. Combine cranberry sauce, ketchup, and remaining herbs; spread over meat loaf. Bake 20-25 minutes or until firm.

Yield: 6 servings.

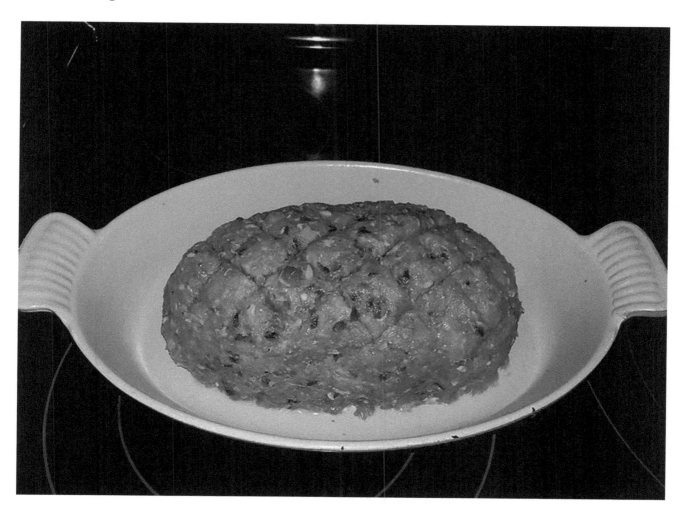

QUICK! HIDE THE BAGS!

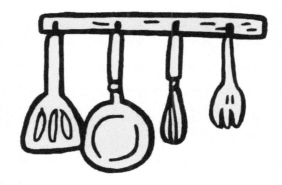

Submitted by David Brock, co-owner of Allprovide Pet Food

We frequently have customers come to our dog food factory enquiring as to why they should switch their dogs from their current, veterinarian-recommended, kibble diet, to our raw pet food. We can take hours patiently explaining all the pros of raw feeding. We educate them about species-appropriate diets, feeding as nature intended, and avoiding highly processed "unnatural" foods. We go to great lengths to show them round our factory. We point out our ingredients, which include restaurant-quality fruits and vegetables and only the best meats, bone and organs. Our philosophy is to feed only the best to all pets.

These potential customers are usually extremely impressed with our ingredients and ethos, and are immediately ready to place an order. This is great...right up until a member of our staff walks into the factory carrying a huge armful of McDonald's meals for our lunches. So much for practicing what we preach for our animals!

In the beginning it was also not unknown for us to work 15 to 18 hours a day; up to our elbows in raw meat, making our raw dog food by hand. Often we were so tired by the time we got home, all we could manage for dinner was a bowl of popcorn and a VERY large glass of wine! Our dogs have always eaten better than us, and still do!

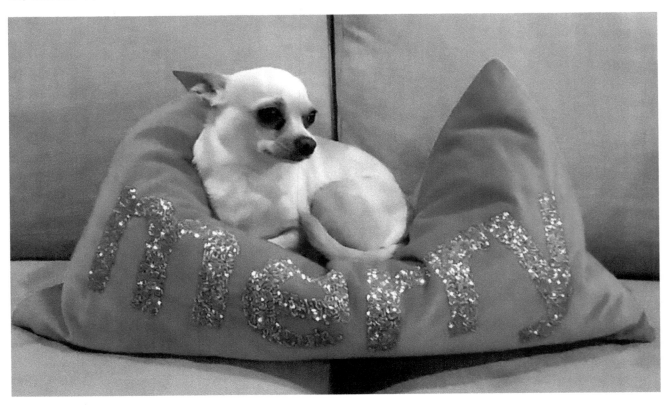

Is this a spoilt little dog or what?

ALLPROVIDE RECIPE FOR DOGS

Look up Allprovide.com

Choose the recipe you want for your dog.

Call and place an order.

Wait for delivery to your front door.

Store in freezer. Thaw as needed. Spoon into bowl. Stand back and watch it disappear.

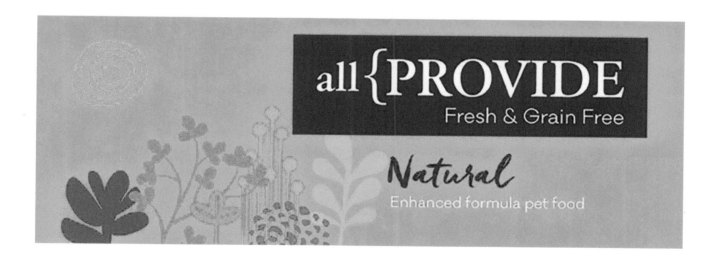

POPCORN AND WINE

Feel free to microwave a bag of store-bought popcorn if you are really tired. But if you want to add a slightly festive touch to your dinner, try these recipes.

Main course: Truffle Oil Popcorn

INGREDIENTS:

4 cups popped popcorn, slightly salted

½ teaspoon truffle oil

DIRECTIONS:

Place popcorn in a large bowl.

Add oil.

Toss popped popcorn with truffle oil.

Take your pick, red or white wine will work with this.

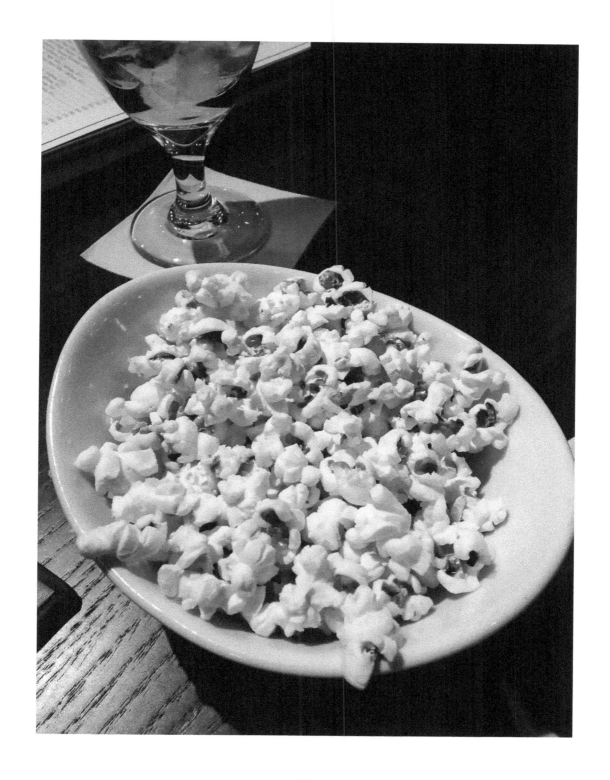

Dessert: Party Popcorn

INGREDIENTS:

4 cups popped popcorn slightly salted

5 ounces white chocolate chips

2 - 3 tablespoons rainbow colored sprinkles (nonpareils)

DIRECTIONS:

Place popcorn in a large bowl.

Place white chocolate in a medium microwave-safe bowl. Microwave at 50% power in 15-second increments, stirring every 15 seconds, just until melted. It usually takes about 1 and a half minutes.

Working quickly, pour melted white chocolate over the popcorn and gently stir until the popcorn is coated.

Top with the sprinkles, stirring to help distribute the sprinkles. Eat immediately if you don't mind sticky fingers. Otherwise:

Spread on a parchment-paper-lined cookie sheet and allow to harden for about an hour. Break up and serve. Keeps up to three days at room temperature when kept in an airtight container.

Should be paired with a sweet dessert wine. According to the Total Wines & More website:

The dessert wine should be slightly sweeter than the dessert itself to achieve the best balance of flavors. A Reisling might be nice, but whatever you have in the house will do in a pinch!

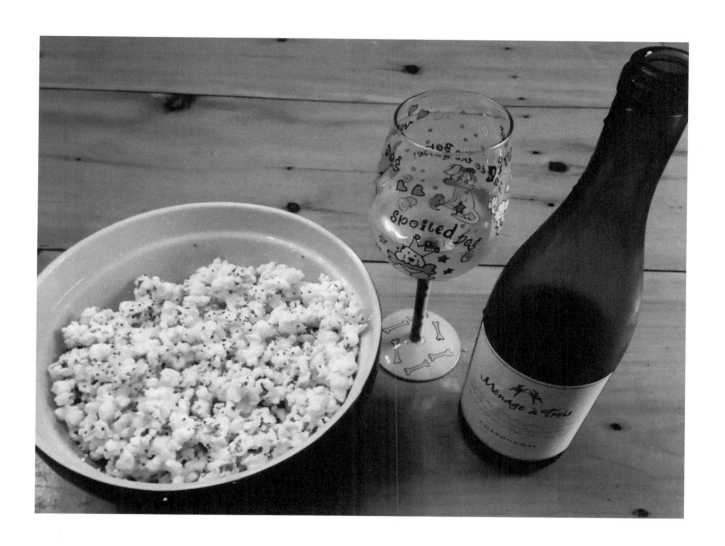

ORGAN MEATS OR STRIP STEAKS?

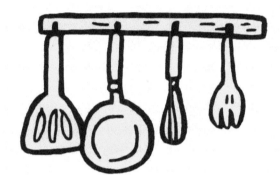

Submitted by Trish Dickinson

From Needles to Natural! Sounded like a book for me and my dog. I'd been searching for ways to make him healthy and stop some of the chronic problems he had been having. How did I get to this point you ask? Here is my story:

Duncan came into our lives 3 yrs ago as a happy, healthy 10 week old, tri- color Cavalier King Charles Spaniel. Being the first and only dog I ever owned, I followed all the recommended protocols. I had him get immunizations at recommended times, neutered at 6 months, applied monthly flea and tick prevention chemicals, and gave heartworm preventative year round. But at 9 months of age, he started going after his foot, growling and biting; the vet kept telling us that Duncan was bored, obsessive, it would pass. At 12 months, we heard the same thing, but my "mother's intuition" told me there was something seriously wrong. After showing Duncan's videos to a group of online friends (Friends of Cavaliers), I really started to be concerned. A visit to the neurologist confirmed an inflammation of his brain. So began our journey that continues to this day.

Throughout this journey, I have had to learn a lot of things, like how to give pills to a pup, dealing with diarrhea as a side effect of the medications, keeping track of his medication schedule, and renewing prescriptions on time, so I don't run out while traveling. I kept trying different foods to test for allergies to stop the itching and inflammation, but nothing seemed to help.

My frustration level rose after months of trial and error. I kept hearing others talk about making "pup loaf", a natural, homemade way to feed your dog. I thought to myself, why not give it a try? Maybe eliminating kibble completely from Duncan's diet would help stop his itching and scratching.

I bought Dr. Morgan's book, found the recipe, and wrote down the ingredients needed: Honest Kitchen base, beef, pork, barley, organ meats...hold up there, organ meats? Where do I get those? Do the stores even sell them? Ugh. I got brave and off to the store I went; looking, browsing, up and down the meat case. Organ meats? What kind of organs? I shuddered to think.

I spied a young man putting out the prime strip steaks. Now, that is my kind of meat! I gathered up my courage and approached him. I couldn't believe I was asking the butcher for organ meats. "Excuse me, do you sell organ meats?" He looked at me like it was an everyday question and led me to the section where I found liver, beef hearts, tripe, and other organs. Who knew those were even available to buy at your local grocery store? I bought up the necessary ingredients and headed for home.

An hour later I found myself squishing raw meat in my bare hands; I don't even like to make my own meatloaf for humans! And another thing...am I the same person who, a few years ago, wouldn't even dream of owning a dog because they were too much trouble?

So began my journey with Duncan on a new path to eating well, in hopes of providing the best I can for him and really, truly hoping he can find some relief with his issues. I know I cannot cure him, but I will do anything (yes even touch, chop and mix organ meats) if I can alleviate some symptoms.

By the way, when I finish making pup loaf, I have no appetite for that strip steak. That's how much I love my dog!

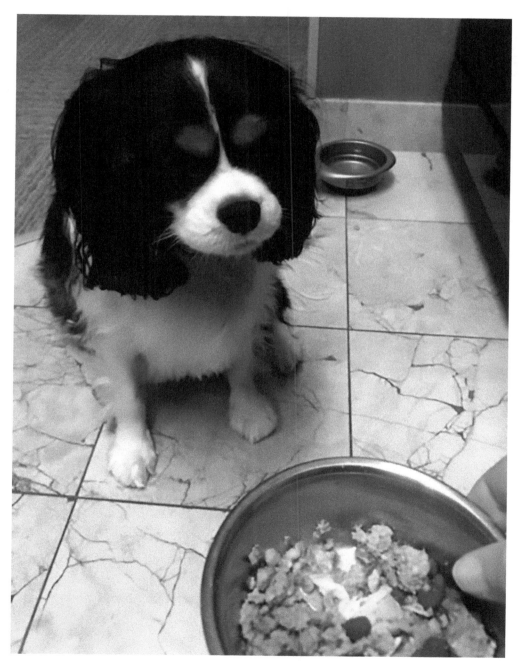

ORGAN MEATLOAF

Submitted by Judy Morgan

10 pounds ground grass fed beef 90% lean

1 pound ground beef heart

1 pound ground calves liver

5 medium carrots

1 cup cranberries

1 cup blueberries

4 ounces Shiitake mushrooms

1 medium size zucchini

1 small bunch parsley

4 ounces spinach

3 stalks celery

2 pears, peeled

2 apples, peeled

1 dozen free-range eggs with shells

1 cup of dry barley (cooked before mixing in)

Grind all ingredients together. We use the metal grinding attachment on our stand-mixer. Mix well in a large pot. Pour into large baking pans. Bake at 350 degrees for 45-60 minutes, depending on thickness. Meat loaf should be moist and juicy. Allow to cool and store in refrigerator for up to 5 days or freeze. Feed about 2 ounces twice daily for a ten pound dog.

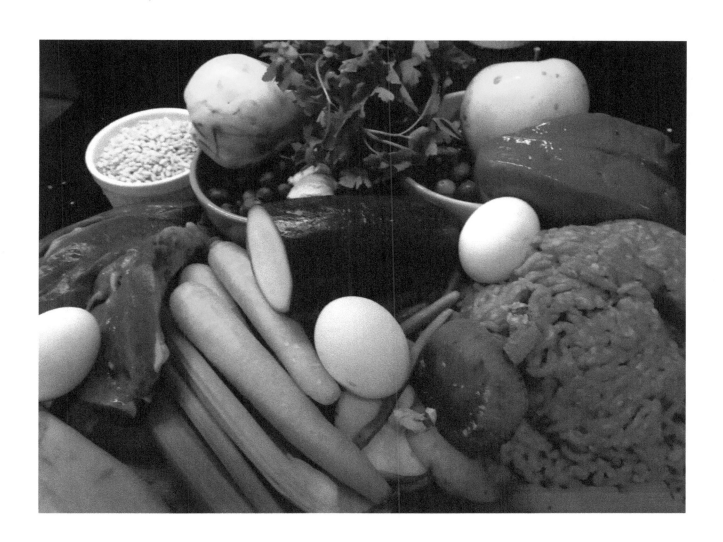

STRIP STEAK

Submitted by Hue Grant

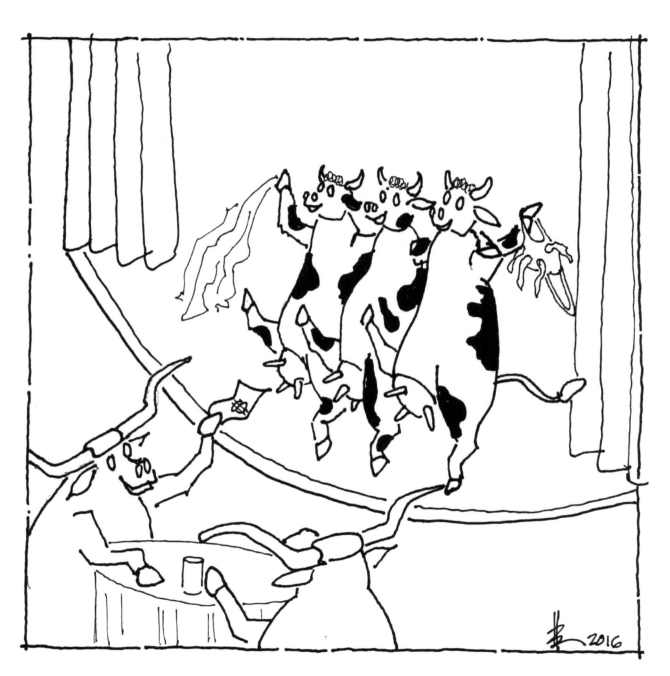

SMORGASBORD FOR DOGS

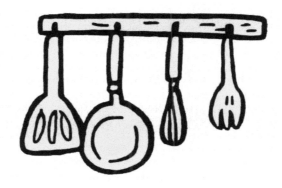

Submitted by Sally Morgan, PetPt
Corgi mom since 1984

I smiled to myself, noticing there was not one vegetable, or even a carbohydrate, in the bags that I was bringing to my vegetarian household. Instead, several heavy canvas grocery bags were filled with ground turkey, ground lean chuck, organic chicken breasts, deli turkey, deli ham, deli Swiss and American cheese, two cans of tuna, and one can of sardines.

Trystan, my young corgi, sniffed the bags from his perch in the back seat, plunging his nose deep into each one. "Sorry sir, those aren't for you. It's for your brother, but you can have the leftovers," I said to him. He patiently sat next to the bags as we backed out of the grocery store parking lot.

Once home, Trystan and I greeted my 16 year old senior corgi, Comet, who barked small woofs and nodded his head in excitement at our return. Trystan gave him a customary lick on his nose. Comet barked back. Comet, unable to move his hindquarters due to degenerative myelopathy, was cushioned on a pile of supportive dog beds, anxiously awaiting his dinner. However, due to the DM and his advancing years, I could no longer predict what would be appetizing to him. He was a grand old dog, and I made every effort to make his meals enticing so that he could keep up his strength. And I really mean EVERY effort.

I began with his usual favorite. "How many years has it been since I have cooked meat in this frying pan?" I wondered, as I turned the turkey burger over to brown it thoroughly. I contemplated keeping this pan just for Comet, so that my vegetarian meals wouldn't taste oddly meaty.

I looked over at Comet, smiling expectantly at me from his thick blue bed across the kitchen. He flapped one front paw at me meekly, waiting to see what I was making for him. Trystan sat like a statue, staring up at the stove, hoping I'd notice how perfectly motionless he was and reward him with some turkey. After adding some thyme, pepper, a bit of salt, and rosemary, I scooped two big spoonfuls of the cooling turkey into Comet's dish.

"Here you are handsome," I said, kneeling next to Comet and offering him the turkey. He surveyed the bowl, took a short sniff, and gingerly lapped up a few morsels of turkey. He squinted slightly and then slowly returned the turkey to his bowl. "Too hot?" I asked him, touching the turkey, which was room temperature. I offered a piece to Trystan who swallowed it so quickly he barely tasted it. I offered another piece to Comet, who turned his head to the side. The turkey went into the refrigerator--maybe for tomorrow?

Back to the frying pan I went, this time adding a spoonful of olive oil to sauté the chicken breasts, adding again thyme, rosemary, and some crumpled sage from the garden. "OK Comet, you'll love this one," I said. As I watched the chicken cooking, I studied the muscle fibers, squeamish after years of being a vegetarian. Scooping the chicken onto a plate, I sliced thin pieces and arranged them in Comet's bowl. Trystan was still a statue staring at the chicken, as I leaned close to Comet, offering him a piece of chicken. He licked my fingers, took a tiny bite of chicken, swallowed, and then pushed my hand away with his nose.

"Still not what you want this evening?" I asked Comet. Corgis are called stubborn, but I see rather that they are persistent and have strong opinions. Comet was politely letting me know that he had other dining preferences. I resorted to the easier foods, opening a can of tuna, one of his old favorites. Singing the bumble bee tuna song for him, I held the can near his nose so he could smell the aroma, as I tried not to inhale--I can't stand the smell of fish. After all, 75% of the taste of food comes from the smell, and with a dog's super powered nose, how could dear Comet resist the yummy tuna? As I approached him with a few bits of tuna in his bowl, Comet flapped his front paws and pushed his body away from the fish. Clearly this was not what he was looking for.

"We are running out of choices here, Comet corgi," I said to him. I rolled a piece of deli Swiss and offered it to Comet. He ate one bite and swallowed. He looked up at me. I returned to the counter and rolled up a piece of American cheese, biting off a little bit as I bent down next to Comet. He sneezed at me. I held the cheese next to him, with Trystan, who finds cheese irresistible, eyeing the cheese, shaking with longing for a bite. Comet refused the American cheese, and Trystan, overcome with cheese desire, snatched up the rest of that piece, slightly nipping my fingers. He looked over at Comet as if he had done it when I looked at him with surprise.

Resorting to the sardines, I rolled back the top of the can the smallest amount possible to remove a single sardine. I held my breath. Trystan's nose twitched curiously side to side at the unfamiliar smell. Comet looked up at me, intrigued. Trying not to inhale, I gingerly put the single sardine in Comet's bowl and slid it close to him. He looked at it, looked at me, looked at it, and looked back at me--a rejection of the sardine. "Well Trystan, this will be in your dinner tonight, when we get to that." Trystan barked loudly, demanding that his dinner come a little sooner, please.

As I browned a small amount of the lean beef, I offered Comet some deli turkey. One bite, two bites, was this what he wanted for dinner after all? Three bites...but no more. I tried the deli ham, one bite. Back to the turkey, no interest. Deli ham, no thanks. "Comet, we are running out of options," I said, fanning the ground chuck in his bowl to cool it off. The beef was unseasoned, as both of my dogs rarely eat beef, and I was no longer certain what to put on it anyway, after years of eating only vegetables. Comet licked the juice from the bottom of the bowl, pushing the meat around in circles, only interested in the liquid. I had to find something he would eat, but what was it? Only Comet knew that answer.

"Shall I fry you some eggs?" I asked him, running out of options as little Trystan followed close behind me, still waiting for his dinner. I pulled out another frying pan, thinking I'd have to buy a whole new set of cook-ware at this rate. I cracked two eggs into another drizzle of olive oil, over easy, planning they could become scrambled in a second if the over easy were rejected. I broke the yolk of one egg and flipped it into Comet's bowl. "Breakfast sir?" I asked Comet.

Again, Comet licked up the yolk, but made no attempt to eat the egg. Becoming desperate, I surveyed the mess in my kitchen, flinging open a window to pull the smell of the meat out of my vegetarian home. Trystan's dish held the rejected sardine, and I added some of the rejected items from Comet's menu. Trystan's favorite food is turkey, so I pulled the ground turkey out of the fridge to add a few scoops to his dinner. As I did this, I heard Comet's little "woof" --"What, so you want turkey now?" I said to him. Growing exasperated, I plopped two big scoops of now chilled turkey into Comet's bowl, after flipping the remaining egg into Trystan's dinner. I set Trystan's bowl on the floor, and he was a very happy little corgi with his mixed up dinner.

I sat on the floor next to Comet with the bowl of recently cooked, and then refrigerated, turkey. I reluctantly picked up a chunk and offered it to Comet. Comet took one bite, and then another, and another, devouring the food completely. I refilled it, and he ate more. Quite satisfied, he licked his mouth and the bowl, looking up at me gratefully. I hugged him, "Oh Comet, I love you" I said, "But I wish you could learn to read a menu so I wouldn't have to cook a million things for you every day!"

Too worn out from the multiple dog entrees I had made, I opened a bag of organic lettuce and herbs from my garden, dumped it on a plate with a splash of olive oil and balsamic, forgoing even the salt and pepper, no signs of nuts or beans for MY protein, and devoured it in seconds. As I wrestled the last bit of lettuce onto my fork, I looked down at sleeping Trystan, eyes closed and tummy full of turkey, chicken breast, sardine, chuck, with some deli cheese and meat to top it off. I could hear the happy breathing of my elderly corgi Comet, snuggled into his puffy blue bed, content with his tummy full of refrigerated sautéed ground turkey. I smiled, realizing that truly I would do anything to keep my corgis happy.

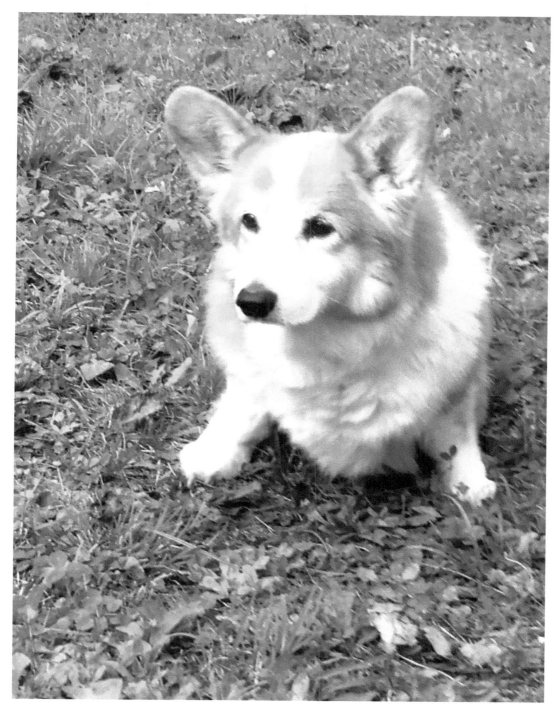

Comet Corgi

FEEDING PETS THAT ARE UNDER THE WEATHER

Submitted by Judy Morgan DVM

Sometimes your dog will be sick or have an illness that may cause decreased appetite. Here are some tricks you can use to tempt your pet to eat.

For upset stomach, brown lean turkey and drain the fat. Mix 2 parts turkey with 1 part organic canned pumpkin. Feed small amounts every few hours until appetite and digestive function return to normal.

Congee is another easy recipe that will soothe any digestive upset. (Including kids and adults!) You can make ahead and keep small batches in the freezer to pull out as needed. To make congee cut up one boneless chicken breast into small pieces (lean turkey or pork can be used if your pet has a chicken allergy). Put in a stew pot with 1 cup long cook white or brown rice. Add 4 quarts water and put on to simmer for 6 to 8 hours. Add water as needed. End product will be a thick gruel.

For dogs with decreased appetite, try cooked sweet potatoes topped with a little cinnamon or honey. Garlic powder or a little crushed fresh garlic may tempt them to eat when mixed with meat. Soft boiled or scrambled eggs are a good source of protein and fat and will provide great nutrition for a dog that is not eating well.

Baby food (without onion powder), cheerios, and dry crackers will sometimes tempt dogs to eat. Although these are not the best foods for dogs, sometimes you have to compromise.

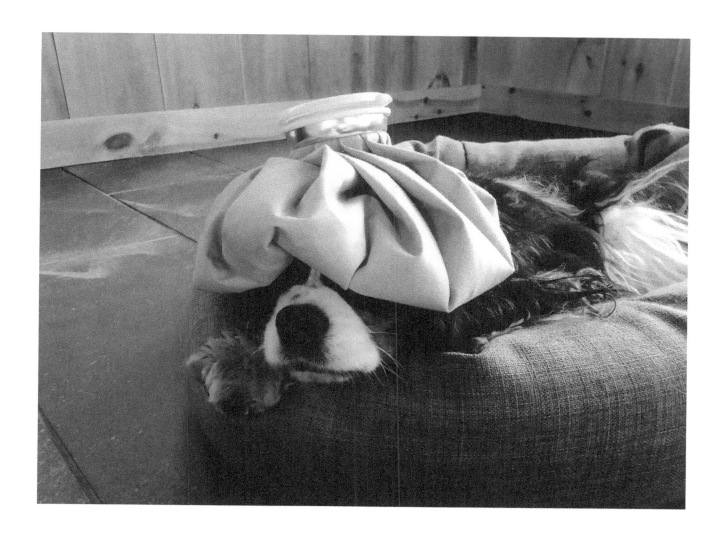

SALAD FOR TIRED PET PARENTS

Submitted by Sally Morgan

When shopping, always be sure to pick up a package of salad mix.

Bonus points if you buy organic. Having tomatoes, cucumbers, snap peas, peppers, or other salad ingredients is optional. You may not feel like adding them anyway.

If you are feeling energetic, mix oil and vinegar in a shaker with some herbs. If not, just pour a little of each on your salad prior to eating.

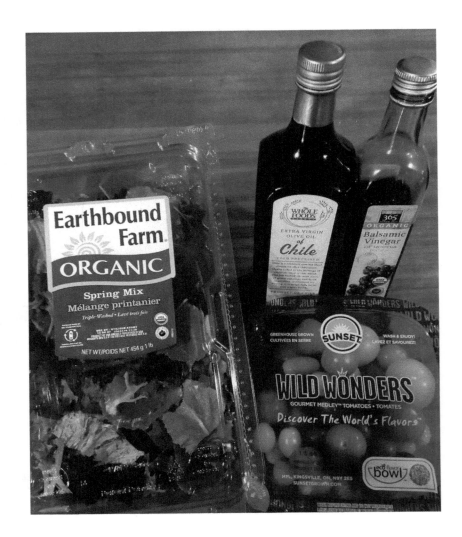

KALE TREATS

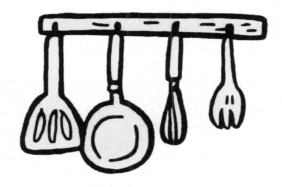

Submitted by Liz Vernon's Lexi and Soldier

Lexi and Soldier here...

Mom made us kale treats! We want more! Mom did this cuz she was reading a diet book. She said she wasn't going to get anymore of those, but Mom is mad cuz according to her Fitbit, she has walked at least 5 miles a day and hasn't lost one pound! Mom even got Dad to get on the weight scale to make sure it wasn't stuck on one number. Well, a lot more than one number, but the same reading.

So she was reading this book and it had all these recipes...including kale treats for her. Mom had already seen a recipe for dogs too, so she decided to do both versions. We got coconut oil and chicken broth on ours. Delicious! Mom baked hers with coconut oil, garlic, and onion powder. She burned the first batch of hers; kale seems to be embedded into her cookie sheet. It's kind of a nice pattern, but she doesn't appreciate that. She didn't burn the second batch, but Mom was making awful faces when she tried it. She says it is definitely an appetite suppressant cuz it is DISGUSTING. Mom thinks she should only cook for dogs, cuz that seems to be the only thing that she can cook. Well, sometimes.

Mom is eyeing her stash of chocolate in the back of the cupboard. Just to kill the kale taste, she says.

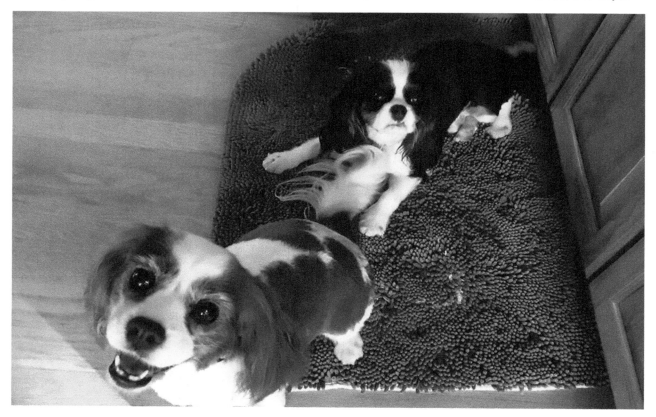

We'd be more than happy to eat your kale chips!

KALE CHIPS TO SHARE WITH YOUR PETS

Submitted by Gwendolyn Campbell

Ingredients:

1 bunch kale, washed and thoroughly dried

2 tablespoons olive oil

Sea salt, for sprinkling

Directions:

Preheat the oven to 275 degrees F.

Remove the ribs from the kale and cut into 1 1/2-inch pieces. Place on a baking sheet and toss with the olive oil and salt. Bake until crisp, turning the leaves halfway through, about 20 minutes.

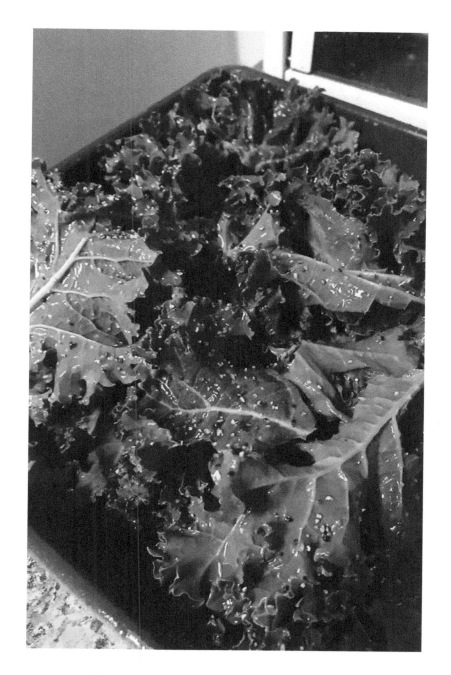

HUSBANDS GET COLD CEREAL

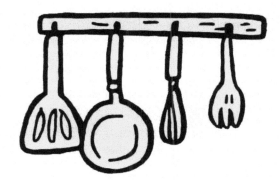

Submitted by Michele Allen, Founder of Monkey's House
– hospice and sanctuary for dogs.

I am a vegetarian and I hate handling meat. The very first Thanksgiving turkey I ever cooked for my family, I didn't cook. When I took the turkey out of the bag and put it in the sink, something didn't look quite right. The neck was still attached. I called my mom, sobbing that it looked like a dead animal, and that I was going to bury it in the backyard. My mom came over and cooked the turkey. I have never cooked a turkey or an entire chicken and I can't eat anything that I've seen whole.

In college I repeatedly asked why I needed three semesters of organic and inorganic chemistry. I gave it my all, and barely got a C in those classes. But what I came to realize, was that it didn't matter what I remembered from those classes; I learned that I could get through things that were overwhelming to me. I've repeated those words several times in my life, mostly in my nursing career, but lately with food prep for my dogs. (But for the record, I still remember that water follows salt in osmosis.)

I've loved animals all my life and have been involved in horse and dog rescue for quite a while. I've always been interested in nutrition for horses, but never found a good source for nutrition for dogs. I spent 18 months home-cooking for a dog that had liver cancer. Even though I didn't know what I was doing, I firmly believe it made a big difference.

I attended one of Dr. Morgan's basic nutrition seminars and started tinkering with my dogs' diets. That three hour class definitely improved the lives of my nine dogs! Nothing had ever come that fast to me; I wanted to learn more. I started taking my dogs to Dr. Morgan. She didn't outwardly say I was crazy when I showed her the allergy dog I had agreed to foster because I wanted to see if I could cure the dog with food. She didn't say I was nuts when I asked her not to touch the second dog I brought to the visit; he bit everybody! (I described him as "not being user friendly".) Instead, she sent me home with some diet tweaks that I was excited to play with.

The changes in my dogs were more noticeable all the time. The dogs were old and sick, but they no longer looked or acted like it. I started noticing certain predictable patterns with my foster dogs. They all came with serious complex conditions and suddenly they were doing extremely well, with fewer veterinary bills.

I had wanted to take my end-of-life fostering to the next level for quite a while, but I wasn't clear exactly what that was or how I would do it. I finally had the answers I was missing! With a tiny bit of gentle, nurturing encouragement from Dr. Morgan (okay, I might have been bullied), Monkey's House, a dog hospice and sanctuary was formed. The sanctuary is named after Monkey, the "not-user-friendly" little dog that I loved so much, who came to me for the last part of his life. It was probably the best part of his life; I know it was an incredible journey for me. The only thing on Monkey's bucket list that we didn't fulfill was biting Dr. Morgan, but that's okay; she helped enhance his last months and he was incredibly happy.

Monkey's House usually cares for 15 to 20 dogs at any given time. The sanctuary is in my home and I spend hours buying, grinding, chopping, and preparing raw meals for the dogs. Sometimes I can spend an entire day working on the project. When my husband, Jeff, comes home from work he can see that the kitchen is a mess and I have obviously been working very hard preparing a gourmet meal. It's really sad to see the look of wide-eyed expectation on his face disappear when I tell him all the mess is from preparing dog food. He will be eating cold cereal...again.

P.S. Until the age of 18, I believed New England was a state between Vermont and New Hampshire.

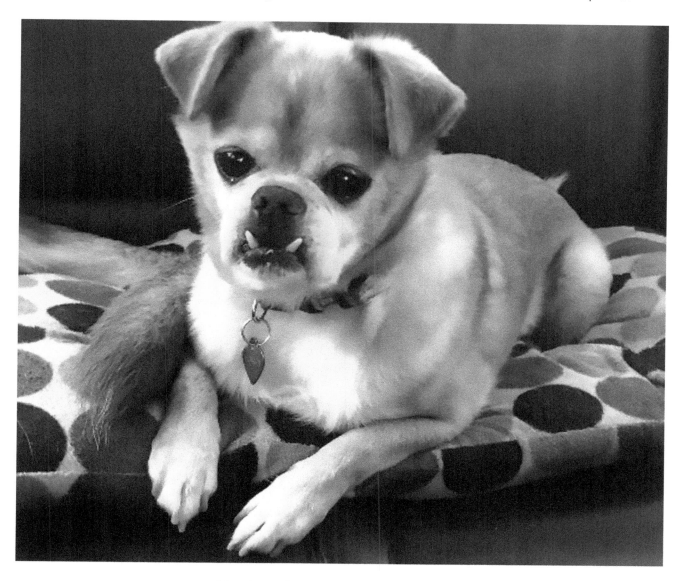

Monkey, the not-user-friendly dog.

MONKEY'S HOUSE HEALTHY SENIOR PUPLOAF

9 lbs free range lean ground beef (90% lean)

3/4 lb ground bison kidney

1/2 lb ground bison liver

1" fresh ground turmeric

6 cups chopped organic kale

14 free range eggs beaten

2 cups organic celery puréed

1" fresh ground ginger

2 fresh turnips puréed,

4 cups shiitake mushrooms puréed

5 cups rehydrated Honest Kitchen Kindly

3 tablespoons finely crushed egg shells.

Combine eggs and rehydrated Honest Kitchen and allow to sit for a few minutes.
Combine the rest of the ingredients and add to egg mixture.
(Make sure husband is available to help place in oven, it's heavy)
Bake at 350 for 1 hr, cool on a slight slant and blot excess fat.

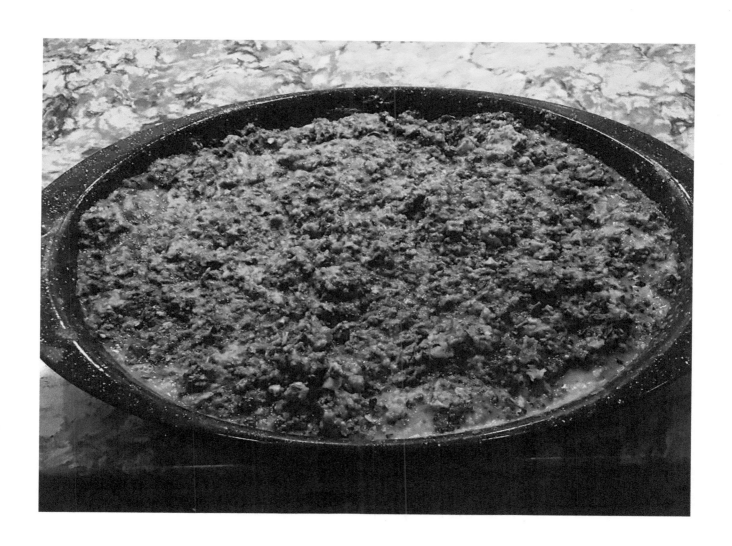

DINNER FOR HUSBANDS

To make the cereal, wash and dry hands thoroughly.

Get out bowl and spoon. Make sure bowl is clean. If not, wipe with your sleeve.

Open cereal box.

Pour cereal into bowl to desired amount.

Add milk if it smells okay. If not, use powdered milk.

Announce that dinner is ready!

(Bonus points if cereal is organic.)

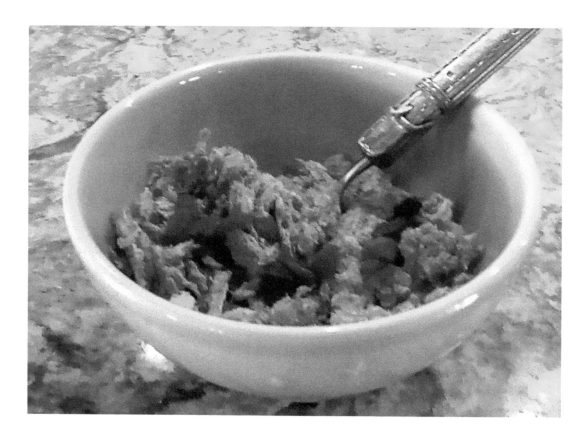

NEEDS SALT...

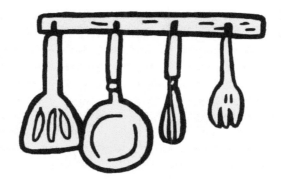

Submitted by Ita Nieves, founder of Beads Fur Rescue

Since becoming a huge fan, friend, and client of Dr. Judy Morgan and following her webinars on cooking for my pets, I've become really good at crock pot and stove top cooking for my doggies. My senior Cane Corso, special needs girl, Lakota, especially benefited from the good, all natural food I would crock pot for her. One particular day I decided to cook up some chicken gizzards and hearts, dragging the stew through the garden with fresh organic fruits and veggies. I added carrots, celery, blueberries, apples, black beans, kidney beans, green beans, peas, sweet potatoes, and topped it off with turmeric when it was ready to be served. I served her portion and then stored the rest in one-cup containers in the freezer.

My husband, who works for the big power company in our state, has to rise and shine with our chickens around 4:00 in the morning to get an early start for work. That morning he decided to just grab something from the freezer to take to work with him for lunch; something he could zap in the microwave and get a warm, home cooked meal. Unbeknownst to me, he just happened to grab one of Lakota's gizzard stews. We usually chat around lunch time and I almost always ask him what he had for lunch. So he called me and I asked him what he had for lunch. He said to me, "You know, I took some of that stew you made the other day and froze in the freezer. The protein tasted different". By this time I knew exactly what he was talking about.

Now you have to know that I am not a big chicken fan, so I don't make many chicken dishes, and gizzard stew for us is unheard of! I started to laugh inside, so I decided to play along. I asked him, "And how was it? Did it taste good?" To my surprise he told me, "Yeah, actually it WAS pretty good! But the next time you make it, it could use a little salt". When I told him it was the doggie's chicken gizzard stew, his reaction was not what I expected; he actually LIKED it! Here I thought he was going to turn green or run to the bathroom...which is probably what I would have done! And there you have it. If it's good enough for people to eat, then your doggies are going to LOVE it!!

Now our new puppy, Tatonka, sits in the same spot her sister Lakota used to, when she waits for her meals. On the stormy night we welcomed her into the family, she waited patiently to be served her first home cooked meal. She continued the legacy of waiting in the same spot Lakota would for her yummy meals.

~Beads Fur Rescue~

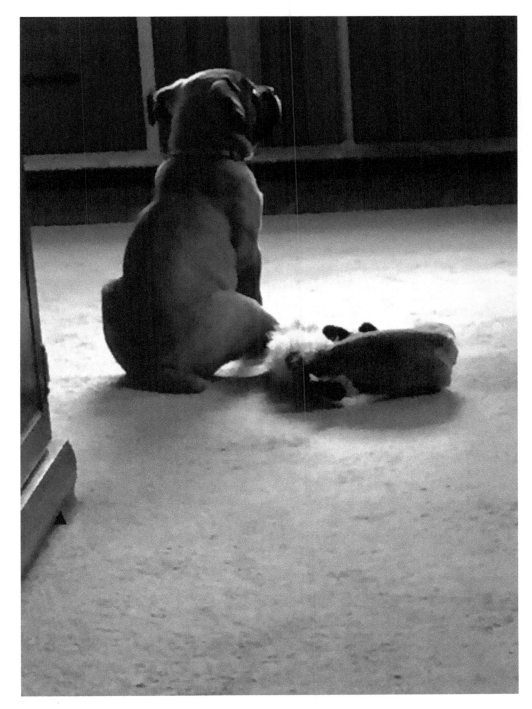

Totonka waiting patiently for her first stew

Chicken Gizzard Stew

Submitted by Ita Nieves, founder of Beads Fur Rescue

Can be shared, but you might want to add salt for humans!

2 packages - frozen chicken gizzards and hearts - cut into small pieces

Fresh organic blueberries - washed and drained

Organic sweet California carrots, peeled and diced

Frozen early peas

Fresh sweet potatoes, peeled and diced

(The veggies and fruits ingredients I add as many or as little as I like or have on hand)

To this you can also add: Peeled diced apples, canned no-salt kidney and black beans (if you don't have no-salt you can just rinse the salt out), frozen green beans, fresh organic celery, diced.

Put all ingredients in crock pot with water covering just to the top. Cook on high for 2 hours then on low for about 4 hours. Serve while lukewarm or room temperature and freeze the rest.

~Beads Fur Rescue~

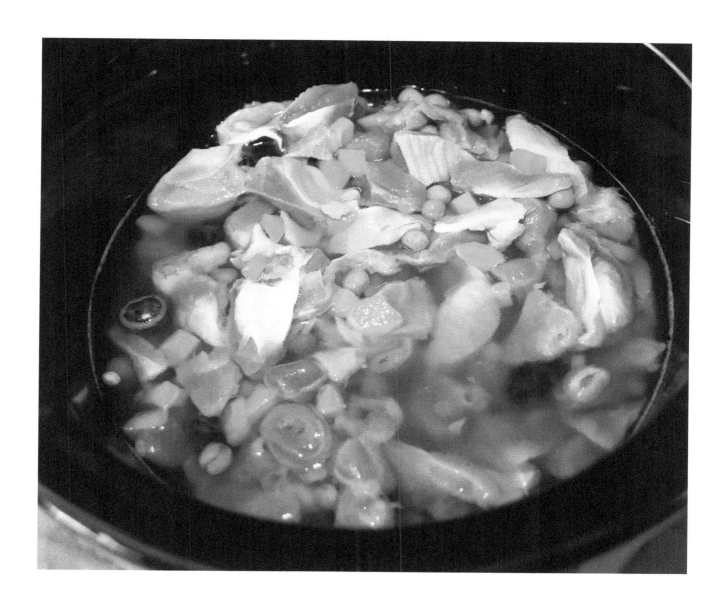

ON THE ROAD AGAIN

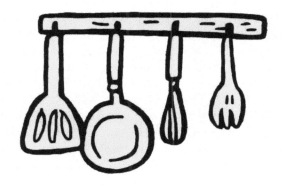

Submitted by Tonya Wilhelm, GlobalDog Training

I consider myself a good dog mom. I understand that nutrition is not only a basic need, but the foundation of my dog's personality, behavior, and energy.

A few years ago, I started home cooking for Dexter, with the guidance of Dr. Judy Morgan. Dexter suffers from syringomyelia, which is a painful spinal cord disease seen in Cavalier King Charles Spaniels. By making meals designed specifically to help decrease his symptoms, I hoped to give him a better life. Home cooking ended up being a life-saver for us on many levels. Dexter has less pain, takes less medication, and has increased energy since I made the switch. Dexter's meals change every twelve days and he has not had the same recipe twice. I use only the freshest, healthiest and most nutritious ingredients I can find. I travel 3 hours round-trip to purchase unusual meats and locally grown organic foods. I order antibiotic and hormone free meats from a reputable distributor online. I don't cut any corners for Dexter; I spend a lot of time designing, prepping, cooking and storing his meals. He is more than worth every second and every penny I put into it.

Me on the other hand...

I try to eat decently healthy food. I look for organic or hormone and antibiotic free foods, but unlike Dexter's meals, I don't require it. I'm a person of convenience when it comes to my own health and eating. If I can't make dinner on a whim in five to ten minutes, I'm unlikely to make it for myself. When I'm traveling, just forget about it! I take coolers packed with Dexter's meals, but gas station sandwiches, muffins, cola, and pastries are the norm for me. I am often harassed on Facebook when I upload my travel meals. People are always telling me just to eat Dexter's meals. I know if I did, I would be a much healthier person, with all my nutritional needs met. But, as the old saying goes, it is what it is.

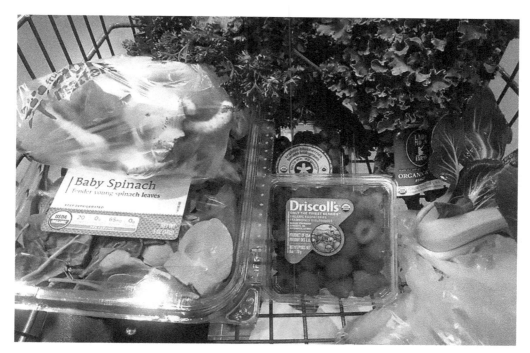

Obviously, these are Dexter's food ingredients!

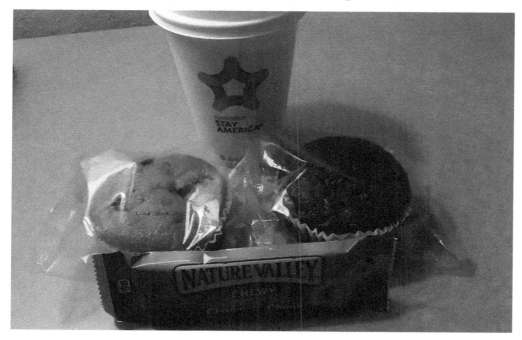

And this is a typical, on-the-road meal for me!

PRE-MADE PUPPINS FOR TRAVEL

Submitted by Judy Morgan DVM

2 pounds of 90% or higher lean ground beef

¼ pound ground beef heart

¼ pound ground chicken liver

2 eggs with ground shells

1 grated apple

1 cup chopped kale

½ cup chopped Shiitake mushrooms

½ cup pumpkin

Mix all ingredients together. Pour into muffin pans. A standard muffin pan will make approximately 4 ounce puppins and mini muffin tins will make 2 ounce puppins. Jumbo muffin pans hold about 6 ounces. One 4 ounce puppin would be an appropriate meal for a 20 to 25 pound dog that receives two meals per day. Keep in a cooler with ice during travel. Can be frozen and thawed before feeding.

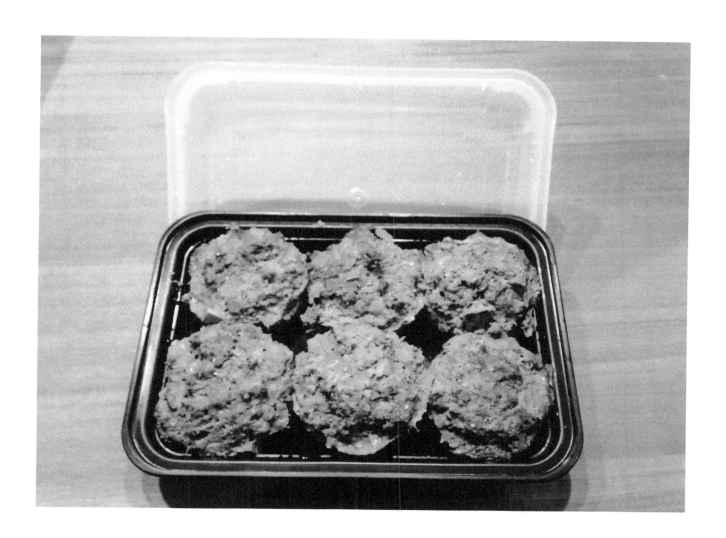

HOW TO EAT HEALTHY WHILE ON THE ROAD

It's impossible.

Pack your own food.

Bananas, pears, apples, oranges, and grapes travel pretty well. Put in a cooler if it's really hot out or the trip is more than one day. Ask your dog if it's okay to share the cooler.

Make a sandwich at home using organic whole grain bread and fresh sliced roasted turkey breast. Add some avocado, lettuce, and tomato. Forget the condiments. They're bad for your health.

Take some organic brown rice cakes for snacking.

Take bottled water and be sure to recycle the bottles.

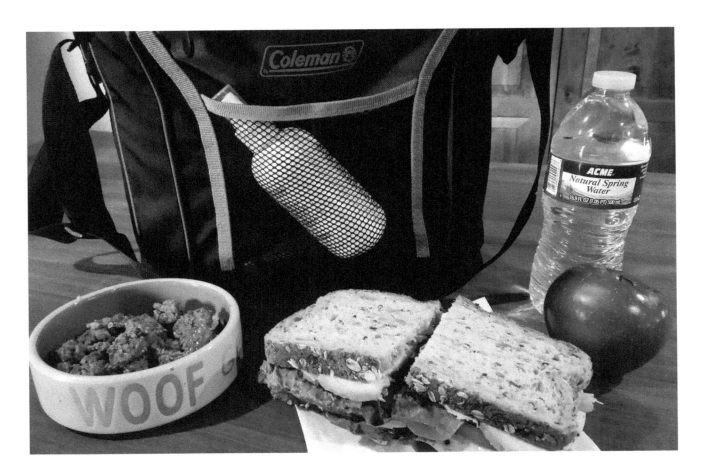

GREEN SLIME

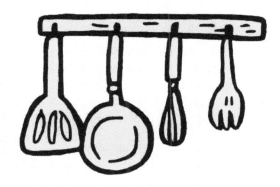

Submitted by Carol Oliver

Making a decision to cook meals for my dogs seemed like a great idea. But I soon came to realize that home-prepared dog food requires me to set aside time to do the preparation and cooking, along with some advanced planning. I buy bulk meats of excellent quality from a restaurant supply warehouse. Eighty pounds of chicken and thirty pounds of ground beef fill the freezer that is dedicated to the dogs. We usually plan a Sunday afternoon to prepare the dogs' food and will make enough for six weeks. We both work together and have perfected our roles and streamlined the process. Unfortunately, I have also come to realize there is a rule that says I will run low or run out of dog food at the most inopportune times.

One Sunday evening, I opened the freezer to discover I was almost out of food. I knew I had a full schedule at work all week and would not be able to find time to cook. The family could live with take-out, but that wouldn't suffice for the dogs. It was impractical to whip up enough food for just one day, so I decided to make a batch of food to get me through the week. Normally I made much larger batches, but I was exhausted and really just wanted to head to bed.

I whipped out my heavy duty food processor to chop the meat and veggies (no time for grinding bones). I thought I would be smart and expedite the process by digging out an antiquated Osterizer blender too. This blender was so old, I had forgotten how to use it. It had been shelved for years. I added a veggie mix to the old blender, turned it on, and turned my attention to my huge meat mix. That Osterizer blender may have been old, but it was fast and powerful.

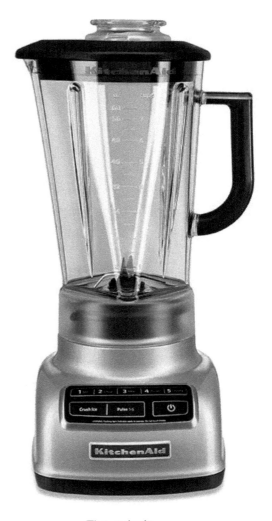

The culprit...

Not even a minute later, I felt a spray of moisture across my back and neck. I thought "I'm so tired it must be my imagination". Then, I felt it again. Then...I saw green stripes across my white cabinets. You guessed it. The seal was not in place in the blender. I didn't think those things would work if not assembled correctly. Apparently, they do, as long as the lid is on. So now, on top of completing the dog food, I had at least 15 white cabinets to clean.

Lesson learned...never begin your dog food when exhausted; plan ahead. And maybe I should have left the old blender on the shelf...

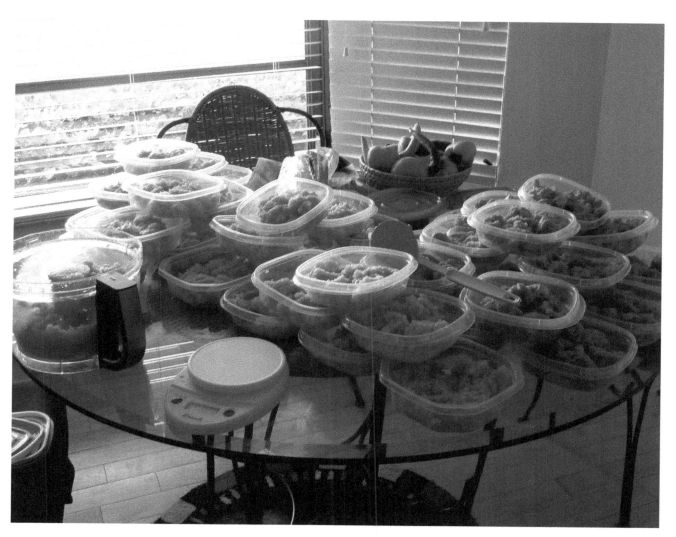

Normal food prep for pups at our house.

RAW FOOD MEAL FOR DOGS

Submitted by Judy Morgan DVM

2 pounds ground 90% lean or higher beef

1/3 pound ground beef heart

1/3 pound ground beef liver

1/3 pound ground beef kidney

1 can pink salmon

3 chicken eggs with ground shell

¼ cup ground carrot

½ cup ground zucchini

½ cup ground butternut squash

½ cup ground broccoli

¼ cup ground parsley

½ teaspoon salt

½ teaspoon ground kelp powder

Feed 1 pound of mixture per day per 50 pound dog. Refrigerate or freeze any excess that will not be fed within 3 days.

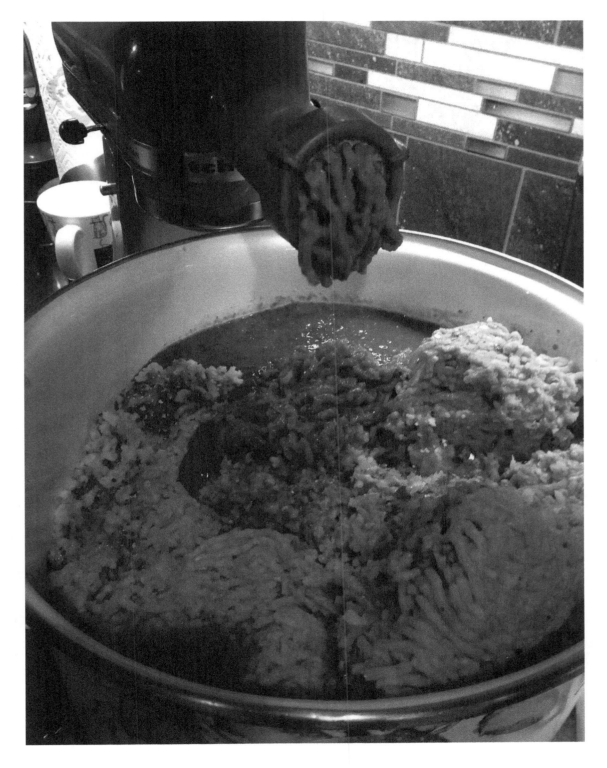

HOW TO ORDER TAKE OUT

1. Decide whether you want Chinese, pizza, or restaurant food.

2. Decide whether you are asking for delivery or pick up. Previous consumption of alcoholic beverages may determine the answer.

3. Look through menus stashed in the kitchen drawer.

4. Whoever is first on speed dial wins or you can call whoever has your credit card on file.

5. Put on pajamas and fuzzy slippers.

6. Tune television to your favorite show or an old movie.

7. Corral all dogs so none escape or eat delivery person when doorbell rings.

8. Eating directly from take-out containers simplifies clean-up.

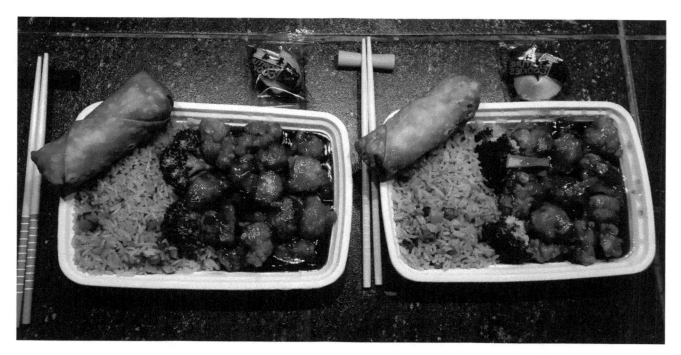

Must be a good day for Chinese food.

MALLETS

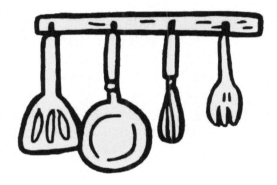

Submitted by Liz Vernon's Lexi, Soldier, and Billy

We really don't like to gossip and we love our Mom, but we are beginning to think Mom is a little well, dim witted. So we are only telling our Facebook friends and maybe a few other people, but certainly not EVERYONE! First, Mom went to a whole bunch of places searching for ground beef heart cuz she is saving for a Vitamixer and didn't have anything to grind with yet. Mom came home with chicken livers, hearts, and gizzards. No beef heart or liver. Then it finally dawned on Mom to call her regular grocery store. They will slice and dice beef heart for her, well actually for us, if she orders it by the case. So Mom orders cases, then realizes she is never gonna fit all that in the freezer. You would think she would have thought of all this in the first place. Mom was determined to go ahead and make our puppy loaves cuz we LOVE these. Mom is amazed someone actually likes her cooking.

So Mom got really ambitious and started emptying some stuff from the freezer to put in our loaves. Ground bison, ground lean beef, honest kitchen, squash, broccoli, green beans, eggs, chicken livers and hearts, sweet potatoes, spinach, and even a shredded apple. Mom was trying to cut gizzards, livers, and hearts and mash up the frozen squash she had defrosted. Mom couldn't find the potato masher and she thinks she might have gotten rid of it cuz she never used it. Dad was downstairs so Mom had the brilliant idea of using dad's mallet. Dad hates it when Mom uses his tools cuz something always goes wrong. Mom washed the mallet and attacked the squash. It was awesome! Squash went flying everywhere! We were even able to lick some off the cupboards and floor. Very cool. Mom even had squash on her face and in her hair. Mom, as usual, had no idea how long it would take to cut up all those gizzards, livers, and hearts into bitty pieces. And Mom kept losing her place in Dr Morgan's cookbook that has the puppy loaf recipe, so she finally held the book open with Dad's mallet.

Mom stayed up til 3am cooking. Dad is a little jealous Mom is doing all this cooking for us and, much to our disgust, she told him we would share with him. Fortunately, Dad wasn't interested. He usually pours catsup all over anything mom cooks, except she is good at meat loaves and soups and that's about it. While waiting for our meat loaves to cook, Mom was reading the cavalier brigade forum and someone mentioned they were up late with 3 cavaliers with gas from having sardines. We already did that and even tho we liked it, she said we are not getting those again because we were emitting toxic fumes. Then someone else mentioned broccoli had the same effect and Mom was thinking she just put a whole bunch of broccoli in the loaves. Then Mom started worrying she might have gotten over ambitious on the ingredients with Soldier's sensitive GI issue.

But the house smelled WONDERFUL! Mom and Dad didn't think the permeating smell of chicken gizzards, livers, and hearts was so great, but we stayed glued to her and Soldier got so excited he did somersaults! Dad wanted to know why Mom had gotten his mallet out for a book weight. Mom mumbled something unintelligible like she does when she doesn't want to answer something. Fortunately, she had already cleaned all the squash off of it. Then Mom started filling the freezer up with puppy loaves and it was more full than when she had been emptying it. See what we mean? Mom can be kind of s-l-o-w in her thought processes.

Even though Mom didn't go to bed til 3 and she's getting sort of old lookin' and she's upset she's getting what she calls "jowls" now, we were ready to go to our favorite place first thing in the morning, the dog park! Dad said it was gonna rain but Mom said it wasn't, so we didn't wear any of our rain stuff. As soon as we got there, the sky opened up. Telling ya, Mom isn't too bright. But that's ok, Mom always keeps towels handy. And we already had our fantastic puppy loaf breakfast. After Mom got us home and all dried off, she asked her neighbor if she could store beef livers and hearts in her freezer that she is supposed to pick up later this week. The neighbor asked if she was now on a high protein diet. Mom said no, she's still trying to stay away from bread and chocolate but really, she cheats all the time.

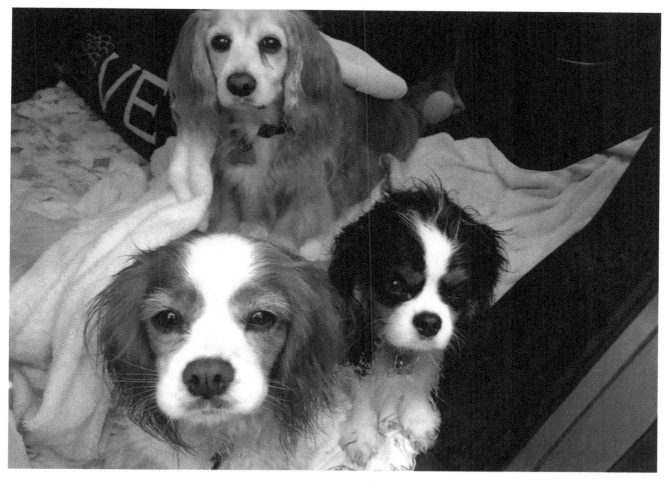

Soldier, Billy, and Lexi

Then Mom started a bleach load in the washing machine cuz she used a whole bunch of white cloths to clean up squishy squash the night before. She threw in Dad's underwear too. Mom didn't notice a red shop rag somehow got in the load and she's turned Dad's boxer shorts pink again. Mom folded them and put them at the bottom of his dresser hoping he will think those are some of those she did that to the LAST time. Mom is now going to take a nap with us and she is simultaneously thinking of chocolate and going to Zumba. There we go again, something not quite right mentally there. Mom always says people will think she is senile when she is 90 just cuz she's 90, but really, she will be just the same as she has always been. But we're thinking maybe that means she's actually been senile all her life.

BUTTERNUT SQUASH BANANA TREATS FOR DOGS

(But you can share if you want!)

Submitted by Judy Morgan DVM

2 eggs

½ cup pureed butternut squash

¼ cup pureed banana

¼ cup honey

2 tablespoons dried milk powder

1 teaspoon cinnamon

Mix these ingredients together. Then gradually add:

2 ½ cups quinoa flour

Roll dough on floured board and cut into shapes with cookie cutters. Bake at 350 degrees for 20 minutes. Flip and bake another 20 minutes or until just brown on the edges. Store in an airtight container and use within a week.

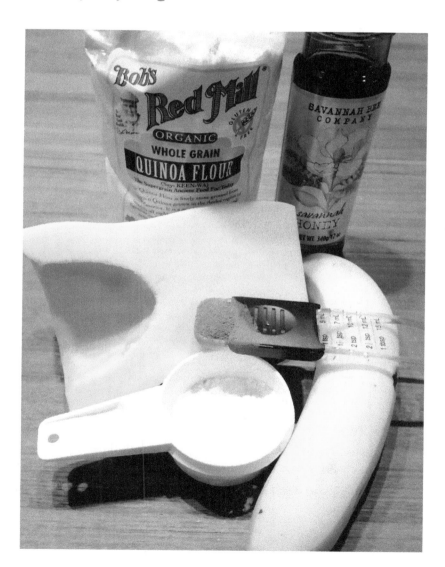

MAPLE BACON PECAN BUTTERNUT SQUASH

Submitted by Hue Grant

Please don't share with the pups.

Prep time: 20 mins   Cook Time: 35 mins   Total Time: 55 mins   Serves 4-5

Ingredients

6-8 pieces of bacon

5 cups peeled and cubed butternut squash (or smashed with mallet if you prefer)

1 cup pecans, chopped

½ cup real maple syrup

2-3 tablespoons bacon fat

½ teaspoon cinnamon

¼ teaspoon salt

Instructions

Pre-heat oven to 375 degrees. Cut bacon into ½ inch pieces. Cook over low heat in cast iron skillet to render bacon fat until bacon is slightly browned. Remove bacon. Let the fat cool in the pan. Combine all ingredients except bacon fat in a large bowl and mix well. Pour all ingredients into cast iron skillet and mix with bacon fat. Use a casserole dish if you do not own a cast iron skillet. Place skillet into 375 degree oven for 35 to 40 minutes or until squash is soft.

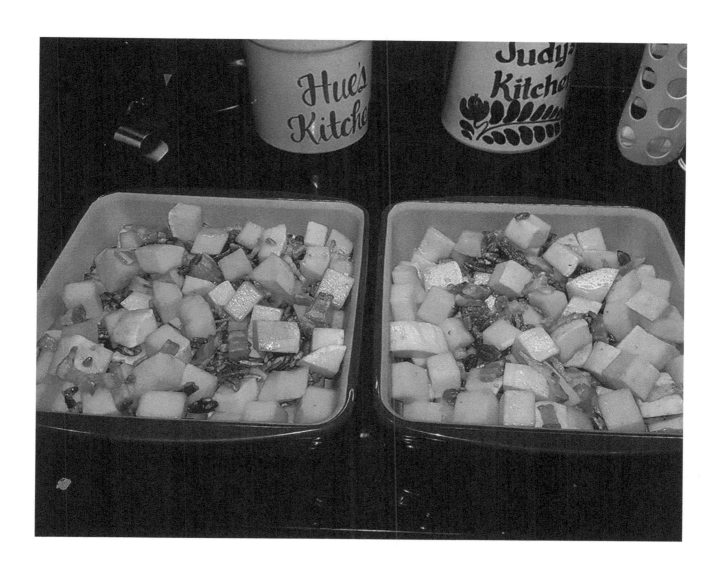

BLOOD TONIC STEW FOR TWO

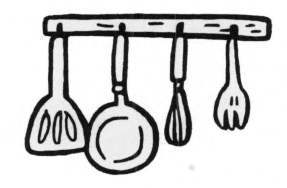

Submitted by Eva Morris

The veterinarian turned to me and said, "I'm sorry there is nothing we can do for Nico. In my opinion I think you should put him down." With a look of anguish and shock, I stared at him and said "Do you mean euthanize him?" His response was just one word. "Yes." I could not believe what I was hearing. I fought the tears, unable to stop the flow. My veterinarian told me if I was not willing to put Nico down, then I should at least give him the prescription dog food and a handful of medications to prolong his life.

But I was not willing to follow his instructions. I decided to do some research and find a holistic veterinarian. I needed to explore what other options there might be. As a result, I frantically searched the Internet to locate a holistic veterinarian that could help me. I came across Dr. Judy Morgan and scheduled a telephone consultation, in hopes of saving my precious dog Nico. She suggested that I home cook and try to help him through food therapy. I purchased her two books *From Needles to Natural* and *What's for Dinner Dexter?* Using the supplements and meals in the books, I managed to keep Nico alive and happy for another 3 months.

As a result of saving my dog, I am now cooking faithfully for my other two Yorkies. For many years I was feeding them commercial dog food which, I now know, was not the best quality. Despite those inviting commercials and enticing photos of healthy dogs on the bag, I now realize that the ingredients leave much to be desired. Some people might feel that it is cumbersome to cook for your fur kids, but I find it enjoyable and rewarding, especially since I feel that they are getting fresh nutritious ingredients and I am in control of the quality of their food. I do not want to be held captive any longer by the dog food industry.

One cold winter evening I decided to make "Chili Dog Blood Tonic Stew". Spanky, my senior dog, has arthritis and trouble with his hind legs, so the "Chili Dog Blood Tonic Stew" looked like a good recipe to help treat his condition. As an arthritic senior myself, I thought I might benefit, as well. I was pressed for time and, since I had quite a bit of beef, I planned on making two versions of the stew; one for the family and one for the dogs. The only difference would be the spices that I would add to the dish that was being served for the family.

I chopped the beef, carrots, garlic, fresh parsley, kale, kidney beans and Shiitake mushrooms. I happily combined all of the ingredients and put them into two separate pots. I added spices to one pot, stirred it well, and went about my business while the chili pots simmered. There was only one problem with my kitchen skills that day: I had a terrible cold and I had lost my sense of smell and taste.

When I was ready to serve the chili that evening, I discovered I had a problem. I could not remember which dish had the spices and which one did not. I couldn't taste or smell anything and now I was in a quandary. What should I do? I did not want to take a chance and have my dogs get sick from the spices that I added. So I did the only thing that a good dog parent would do. My family was going to get both dishes! Luckily, I had some pup loaf sliced in the freezer, so at least my dogs would be eating that night.

I quickly packed away one version of the chili and froze it, as I served the other one that I had left. I did not want my family to know that they might be eating the dog's food! I have already been through the meatloaf questionings of "Is it or isn't it our food?" or "Is that for the dogs?" Since I put so much love and effort into making food for the dogs, I think my family should feel honored to get the dog food.

As I sat and watched everyone eat the chili, I could not help but wonder if it was the one for the dogs or not. "So how is it?" I timidly asked. "It's good but it tastes very bland" my husband responded. I quickly went into the kitchen and got some chili, cumin, oregano and garlic powder and told him to add some more. I used my cold as an excuse, but he just clarified to me that he was pretty sure he was eating the dog's food and the chili in the freezer was actually the meal meant for the family. To this day, it is my little secret and they will never know that they ate the "Chili Dog Blood Tonic Stew". My mental wheels are turning now as I thumb through the book to find another recipe that I can cook for both my family and fur kids.

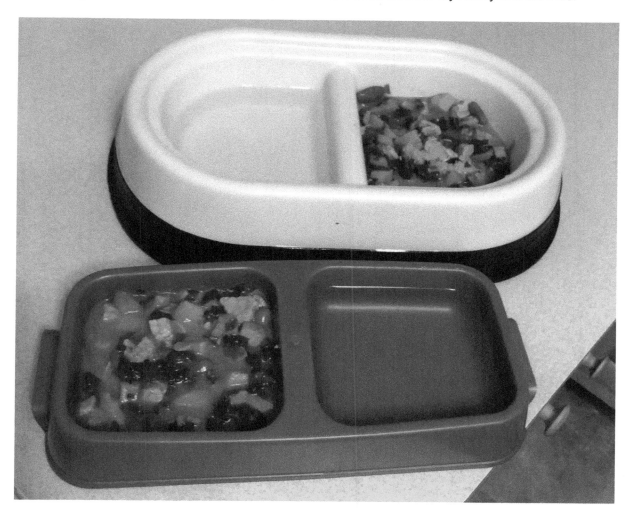

CHILI DOG BLOOD TONIC STEW

(Modified)

Submitted by Judy Morgan

5 pounds beef cut into small cubes

1 pound beef liver

5 cups kale chopped

3 cups spinach chopped

4 cans sardines in tomato sauce

6 ounces canned crushed tomatoes

5 large organic carrots peeled and chopped

5 cloves fresh organic garlic peeled and crushed

1 bunch fresh organic parsley chopped

2 cans organic low salt kidney beans

1 cup chopped organic Shiitake mushrooms

Put all ingredients in a slow cooker or heavy pot on the stove. Add water to cover the ingredients. Cook all day.

Not all dogs digest kidney beans well. If you know your dog does not do well with beans, 1 cup brown or wild rice would be a good substitute.

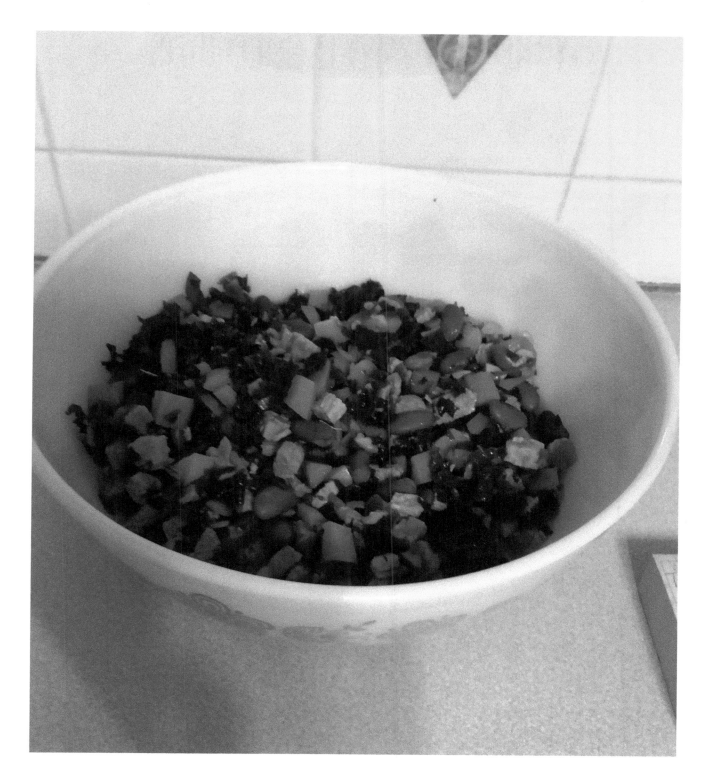

CHILI FOR TWO-LEGGED KIDS

Submitted by Hue Grant

1 and 1/2 pounds beef cut into small cubes

2 large onions peeled and diced

2 red bell peppers cored seeded and diced

16 ounces canned crushed tomatoes

2 cans organic low salt kidney beans

2 cups beef stock

1 12-ounce can of beer

3 cloves fresh organic garlic peeled and crushed

3 tablespoons minced fresh ginger

2 jalapeno peppers cored seeded and minced

¼ cup olive oil

¼ cup ground cumin

¼ cup ground coriander

¼ cup paprika

1 tablespoon ground cinnamon

1 tablespoon curry powder

Brown the meat in a small amount of olive oil. Pour off the fat. Set meat aside. Add remaining olive oil. Add onions and peppers, stirring occasionally until they begin to color (9-11 minutes). Add garlic, ginger, and jalapeno peppers. Cook, stirring constantly for 2 minutes. Add remaining spices and cook, stirring, for 3 minutes more. Return meat to the pot, add kidney beans, beef stock, and beer. If there is not enough to cover all the ingredients, top off with more beer. Bring to a simmer and skim any scum off the top. Cover, reduce heat to low, and cook for an hour and a half or until meat is tender.

While cooking, feel free to partake of the remainder of the six pack of beer.

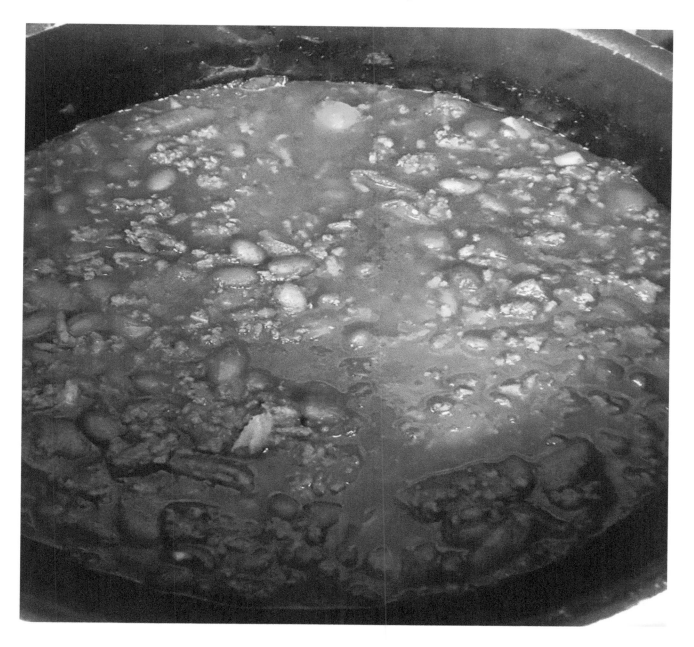

BAND-AIDS

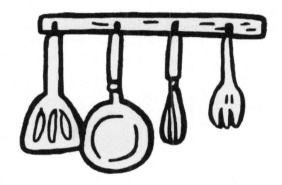

Submitted by Liz Vernon's Soldier, Billy, and Lexi

Mom is at it again. We know we told on her before about her being a little dimwitted, but did we mention that she is accident-prone? Mom got good advice from Aunt Janet who suggested a $60 Ninja on e-bay instead of saving for a Vitamixer and Mom is delighted with it. Aunt Janet warned her that the blades were sharp. She did. First thing mom did was slice her finger assembling it. Mom already had a band-aid on from getting stitches on her thumb last week (different story) and mom had to put another band-aid on cuz she was dripping blood all over the Ninja instruction pamphlet.

But Mom managed to get the Ninja put together and ground the beef heart and added it to all the other good stuff and pureed the beef liver with the pumpkin. That was with 8 pounds of bison and ground meat, broccoli, green beans, Honest Kitchen, blueberries, and a bunch of eggs. She said if she was going to cook, she would rather do a whole bunch at once. Mom even used a regular paperweight on Dr. Judy Morgan's cookbook this time instead of Dad's mallet. We were sorry she didn't use that again. But all was not lost. Mom also simmered some beef livers on the stove for us separately.

Mom was so happy that she was not going to stay up most the night this time because of the Ninja now doing the grinding. But just in case, she started our food production this morning. Mom got it all mixed together in this huge industrial bowl and just as she finished, she realized she had lost the band-aid. Mom panicked, thinking she lost the band-aid in the meatloaf mix. Mom kept squishing portions to find it. Then she tried taking small balls out and squishing that into another bowl to find it. Mom was getting really worried. So then she took a ball at a time and spread it across the cutting board. Still, no band-aid. Mom then went out to the garbage bag she had taken to the canister outside and emptied all the garbage, searching for the band-aid. She didn't find it. Mom came back and did another round of flattening portions on the cutting board searching for what she was now calling the *?!%* band-aid! Dad walked in then and wanted to know why she was flattening meatloaf guts on the board. When Mom explained, Dad said we couldn't eat a band-aid; that would be really bad. Mom glared at Dad. He went downstairs to his man cave.

Mom decided she would have found it if it was in there, but it still bothered her. She made so many loaves she had to do 2 rounds in the big oven. Cool! Since Mom is always dropping things, we stayed close. Billy always takes the prime position in the center of the kitchen to watch for flying treasures.

While the first round of meat loaves was in the oven, Dad walked in again and asked what that smell was. Mom had completely forgotten the livers on the stove during her band-aid panic attack. They were rubber. Dad decided they could be bounced. So he bounced one and we all went nuts trying to get the bouncing liver! It was so much fun!

Mom got the first round out of the oven, and Dad walked in again. Dad wanted to know why they looked kind of purplish-gray. Mom said she had added a bag of blueberries. Dad said he didn't think she should have added a whole bag. Mom glared at Dad again and he exited for the man cave again. Good move.

WE had a great dinner tonight, even though Mom made the meatloaf into meatloaf crumbles in our bowls; she's still fixated on that band-aid. Dad has requested that Mom start marking dog food in the fridge and the freezer because he's afraid to get anything out of the fridge or freezer now. He thought he was getting human meatloaf last time he pulled one out. Don't know what his problem is...

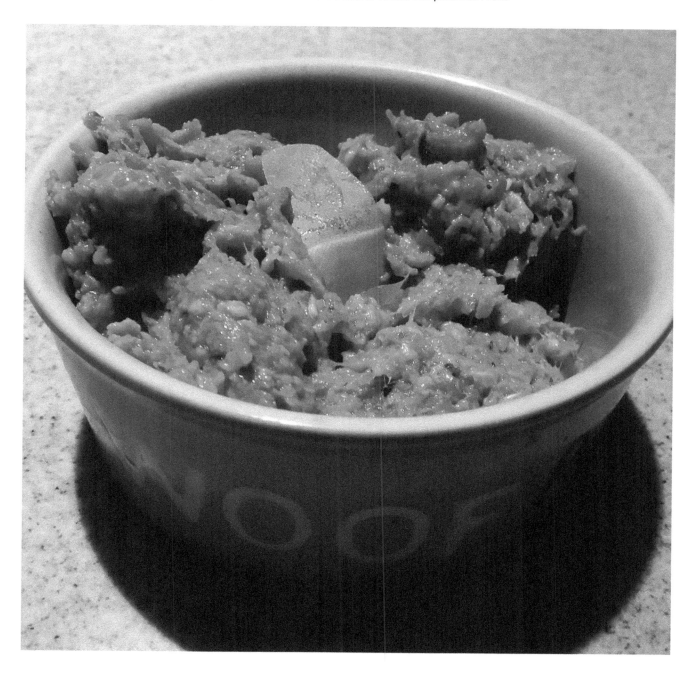

BAND AID-FREE PUPLOAF

2 pounds ground bison

1 pound ground 90% lean beef

½ pound ground beef liver

½ cup chopped broccoli

½ cup chopped green beans

1 cup pureed pumpkin

3 eggs with ground shells

½ cup chopped kale

¼ cup chopped Shiitake mushrooms

Combine all ingredients. Mix well. Pour into loaf pans. Bake at 350 until firm, usually 45 to 60 minutes, depending on size of pan. Should be a bit underdone rather than overdone. Feed 4 ounces per 20 pounds of body weight twice daily.

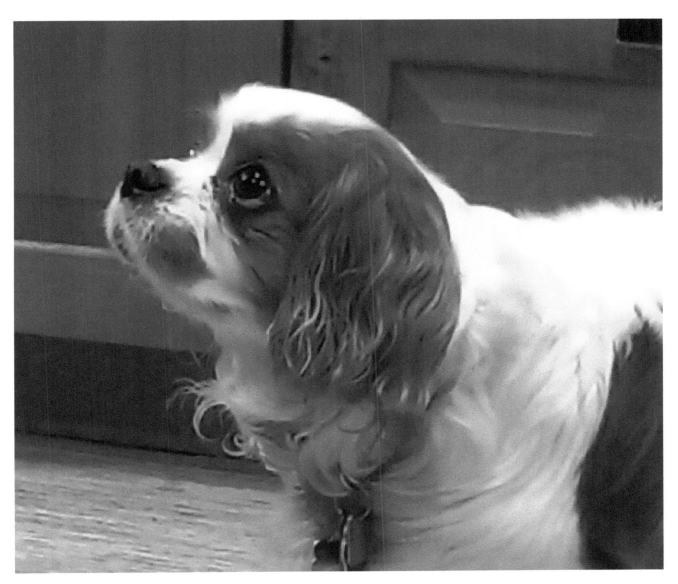

"Can it cook any faster please?"

BISON MEATLOAF

Submitted by Hue Grant

2 pounds ground bison

2 eggs beaten

1 Tbsp. Extra virgin olive oil

1 Tbsp. unsalted butter

3 cloves crushed garlic

¼ red bell pepper chopped

2 stalks celery chopped

¼ sweet onion chopped

½ cup panko breadcrumbs

½ teaspoon black pepper

½ teaspoon salt

2 teaspoons Worcestershire sauce

½ teaspoon fresh ground thyme

½ teaspoon fresh ground oregano

½ teaspoon fresh ground rosemary

Sauté garlic, red pepper, celery and onion in olive oil and butter until translucent and allow to cool. Combine sautéed veggies with the rest of the ingredients, form into a loaf and place on a rimmed baking sheet. Bake in 350 degree oven for approximately 60 minutes.

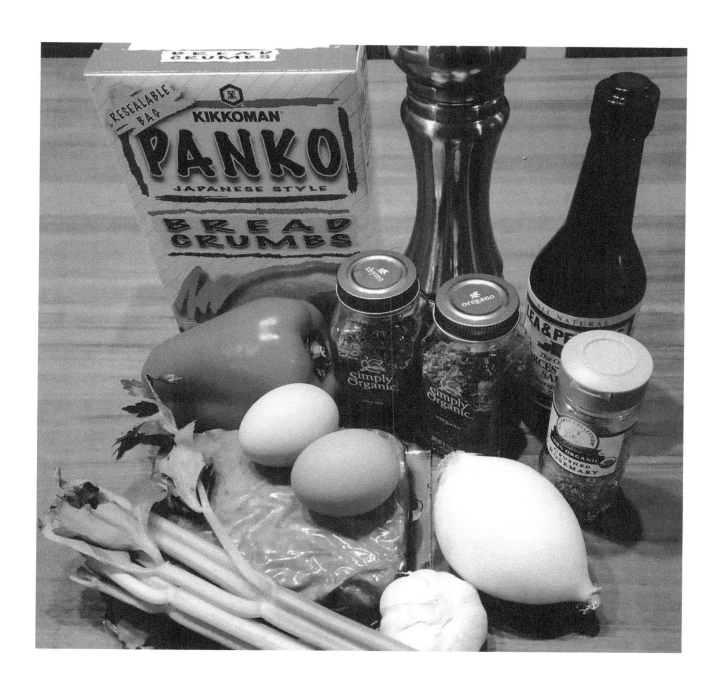

BE PREPARED

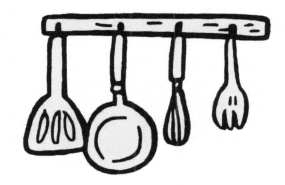

Submitted by Kristy Hess

I am a Girl Scout leader and the motto "Be Prepared", rings true in my life, as I believe in being prepared. I took a course and became certified in home canning so that my family would always have food available in an emergency. Of course, this also comes in handy for everyday use, as home canned foods are so much healthier than any processed food I could purchase. There are safety rules I must follow in canning and I make sure that is always foremost in the process.

One of the most precious members of my family is Bella, an adorable little Chihuahua. Bella is a bit lazy and really could stand to lose a pound or two. She is very content to be a lapdog, but I knew she would have more energy if she was eating healthy, home-made food instead of processed food. After reading *What's For Dinner Dexter?*, I thought, why not find some recipes in the book that could be safely canned for Bella? I knew I could can in small sizes just right for her. After all, she should have her own shelf, stocked with stable, healthy, home-canned food, ready to go in an emergency. So, I found several recipes in the book that I thought would provide her with the right blend of nutrients and help restore some of the youthful energy she once had.

I found many recipes with no flour, grains, or dairy, which are three ingredients that should not be used in canning. I found a great deal on chicken, so I modified one of the diets to use chicken instead of turkey. I used an eighteen-quart electric roaster and multiplied the recipe by thirty. One problem with the recipe was the use of organ meat, which is not approved for home canning due to density issues. I solved the problem by grinding up those ingredients, combining them with other ingredients, and adding sufficient water to process. The density issue was eliminated.

Bella was very interested in the process taking place on the counter above her. Her little nose worked overtime while she sat under my feet. But she had to wait another day, as the canning takes a little more work than just making the stew. The next day I had to process the jars in the pressure canner. The chicken needed to be processed for ninety minutes at ten pounds of pressure. The three batches took me close to three hours each. Bella was on high alert, right behind me the whole time. But eight to nine hours of love for my dog resulted in sixty seven, individual, shelf-stable meals for Bella! The ingredients cost a total of $32.50, which works out to about forty eight cents per jar. That's about one third the cost of buying "high end petite meals" from the pet store that contain ingredients I can't even pronounce.

So, after two days of shopping, cooking, and canning, there was no time left to cook a good meal for the humans. They got hot dogs. Bella had her first plate of her home cooked food made by "Mommy". She wagged her tail in approval as she dined, totally uninterested in our hot dogs. Normally she would have been begging for those hot dogs, instead of eating the processed food she had been served. Now she barks for her food!

This was totally a labor of love. Knowing what was going into Bella's food, and that it was processed safely, made up for the time I spent preparing her meals. Bella knows what's in it too – stuff she likes! The ingredients are also specific for her needs, as there is no one-size-fits-all diet. I'm looking forward to canning a beef recipe next. Bella's meals now take up much more space in the canning pantry, but with all the money she is saving, she can buy new clothes. Yes, she likes to dress up!

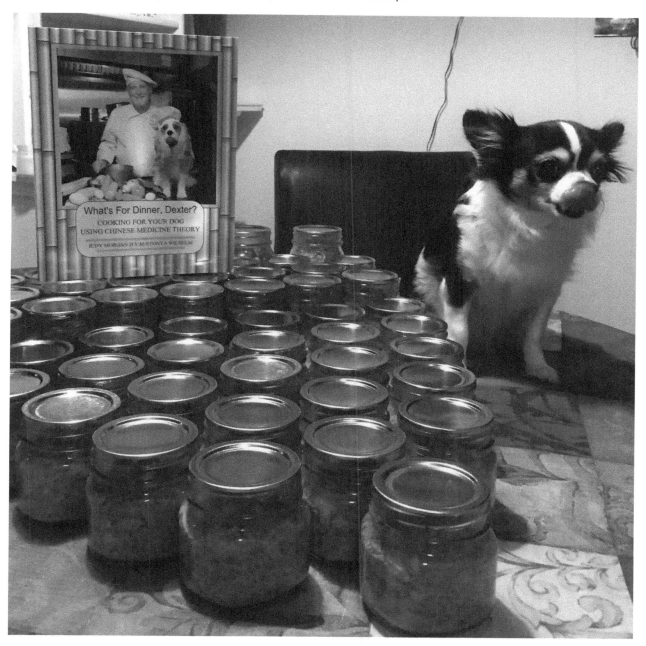

Bella says "Mine, all mine!"

CHICKEN STEW FOR CANNING

Submitted by Kristy Hess

16 ounces Chicken Thighs, Boneless, Skinless

16 ounces Chicken Legs, Boneless, Skinless

12 ounces Beef Kidney

6 ounces Turkey Hearts

6 ounces Sweet Potatoes

1 Apple

1 Banana

3/4 cup dry Green Lentils

Wash and peel the fruits and vegetables; cut into bite-sized pieces.

Cut the meat into 1" chunks.

Place all the ingredients into the slow cooker. Add enough water to cover the food.

Place the lid onto the pot, put on low, and simmer for 8-10 hours.

When finished, cool and proceed with canning process, or put in freezer-safe containers.

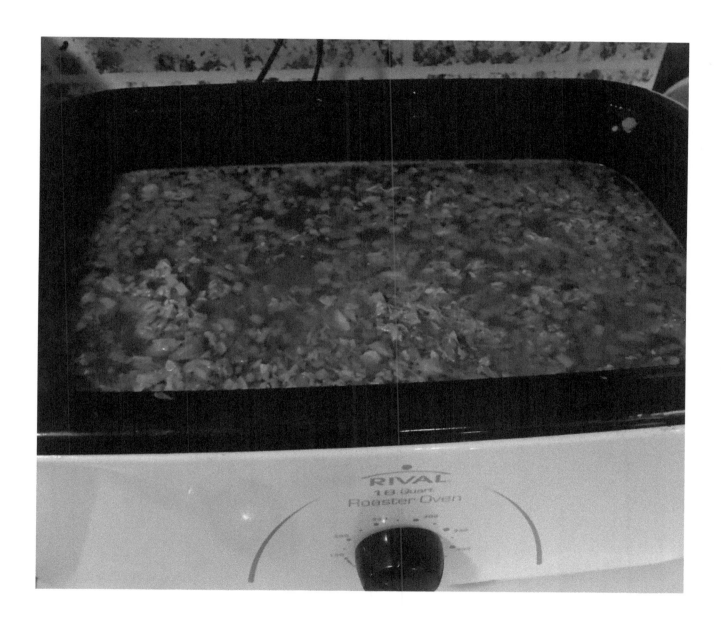

HOT DOGS FOR HUSBANDS AND KIDS

Prepared and submitted by Hue Grant

The family will think you went a little too far chopping meat with these ghoulish hot dog fingers! Remove a small circle of meat for the fingernail and make slashes across the knuckles before boiling. Serve with ketchup "blood".

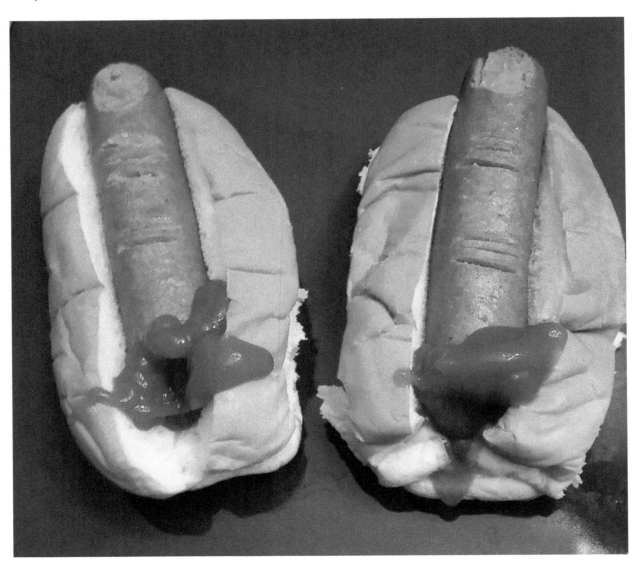

Yup! Hot "dogs" for humans. Wrap hot dogs in Pillsbury Poppin' Fresh dough sheets leaving extra at each end to form head and tail. Form feet and ears out of dough. Bake according to directions on dough container. Add cheese circles for the eyes and Juniper berries, ketchup dots, or peppercorns for the eyes and nose.

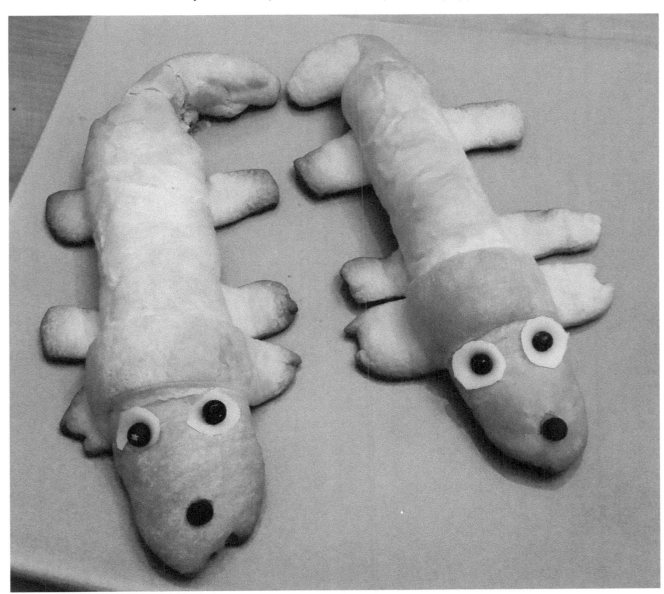

Make hot dog "Octopus" by inserting four long spaghetti noodles through a piece of hot dog before cooking. Boil in water until pasta is soft and hot dogs are cooked.

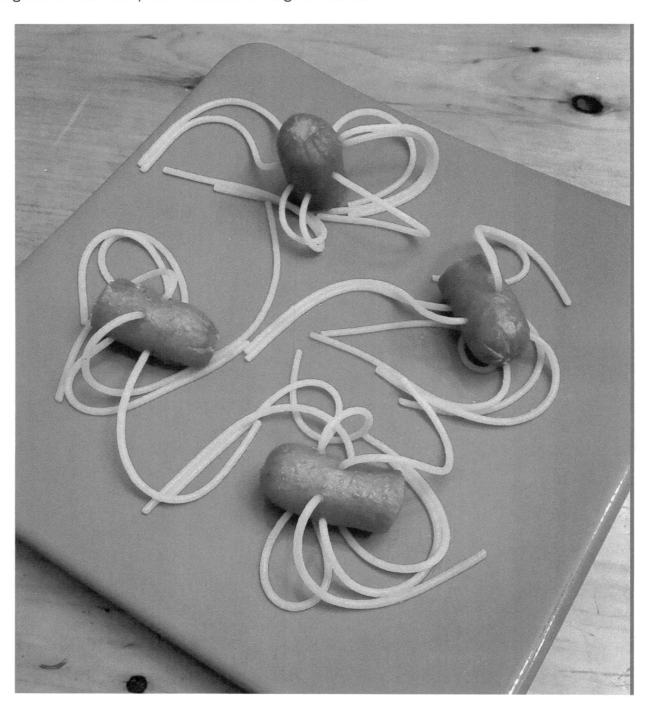

Every dog deserves a dog! Use a hamburger bun, cooked hot dog, and cheese to make ears and eyes. Nose and eye centers can be Juniper berries, ketchup, or peppercorns.

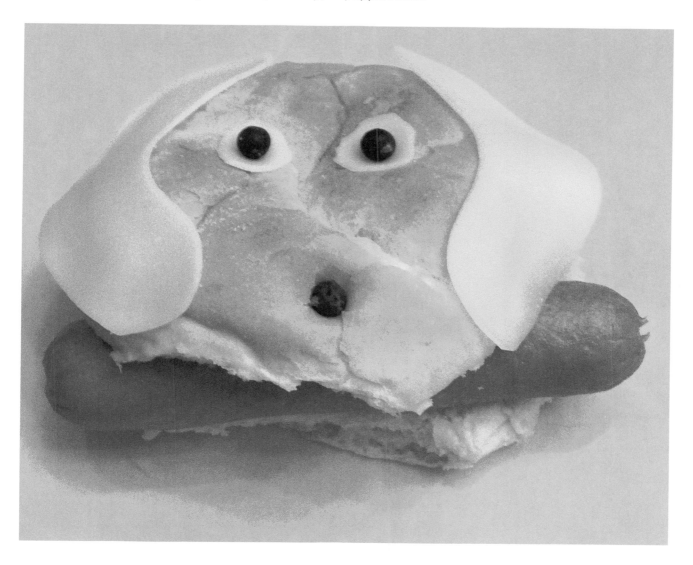

Delicious mummies! Wrap strips of dough around the hot dogs and bake in the oven for ten minutes. Add mustard eyes.

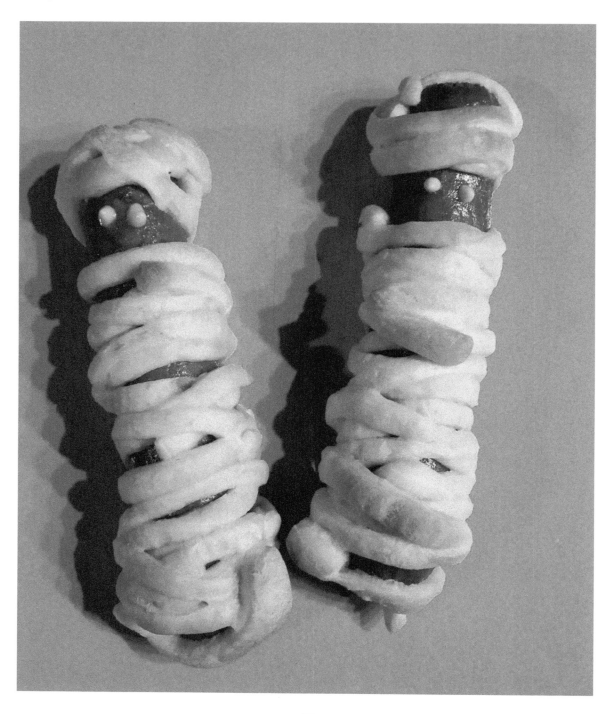

If you are really tired, just boil the darned hot dogs, throw them in a bun, and offer ketchup or mustard as the only choices.

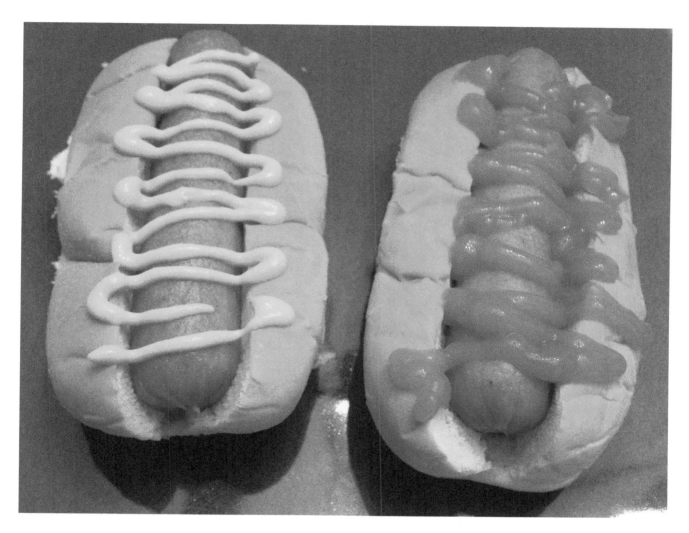

BLUEBERRY PROBLEM

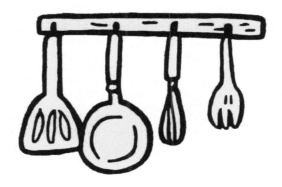

Submitted by Liz Vernon's Soldier

Soldier here...I'm doing a solo speech cuz Lexi and Billy are nodding off. I'm plugged. Yes, plugged. Mom got a little overconfident adding ingredients to the puppy loaves. Mom actually said "a little too cocky", but I'm a little more polite than that. It was either the pumpkin or the blueberries, or both...but we liked eating it! That's why Billy and Lexi are nodding off...they had what you might call an "exerting" day. At least they exerted. Mom made us an interim simple loaf and that got their systems going.

But enough about that subject...we live in a retirement community and what is it about some elderly people that have to tell Mom all about their bowel, um, activities? Mom is vowing not to do the same thing when she gets older. But you know, she's the dim witted one...first she wasn't thrilled she was the youngest one around...now she's not thrilled she's starting to look like she blends in. Mom better remember all the things she is grateful for...like us! And I'm the one that has the, uh, PROBLEM. So tomorrow, Mom is going to make some more simple puppy loaves for us and skip pumpkin and blueberries.

Meanwhile, she is dismayed she still has 11 loafs of the plugging stuff in the freezer. Any non-dimwitted person would have realized new ingredient experiments should have been done in small batches. And THEN, Mom is going to make Dad some human meatloafs cuz he keeps complaining we get meatloafs and he isn't getting any. Oh...perhaps that last sentence should have been worded differently. I'm talking about MEATLOAF, people! Mom says she might as well open a meatloaf production factory. Without pumpkin, blueberries, and no band-aids again, ever!

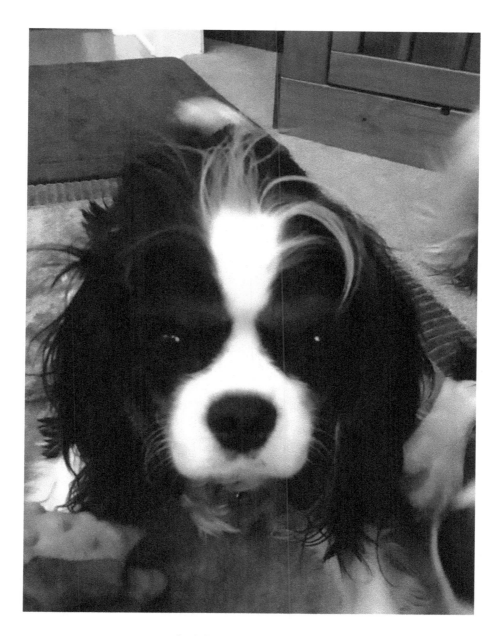

Soldier, reporting in.

FRUIT SALAD

Can be shared with humans or dogs.

Cut up your choice of melons, pineapple, mango, papaya, bananas, and berries. Please do not use grapes or raisins in your recipe.

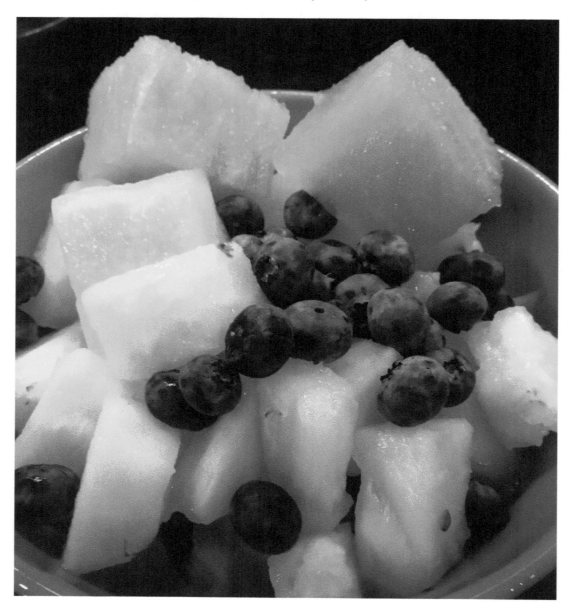

ONLY THE BEST FOR
THE LADY OF THE HOUSE

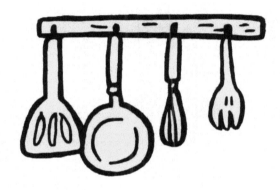

Submitted by Deborah Heidt Cordone

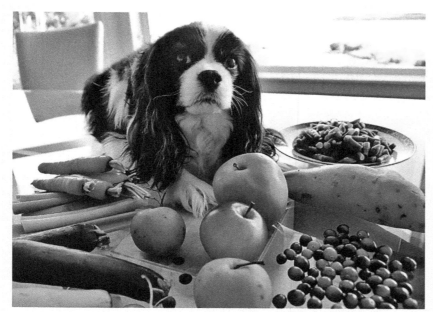

DOG FOOD ◀

BAD FOOD ▶

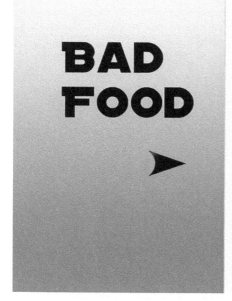

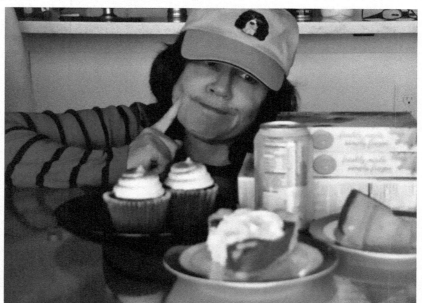

Decisions, decisions...

My beautiful Lady C, a tri-colored Cavalier King Charles Spaniel, just celebrated her 10th birthday. She has been with me since she was 10 weeks old! Lady C is a bit of a canine celebrity since she authored her own book *Pawsitive Reflections*, which we published to raise funds for cavalier rescue (though she is not a rescue herself). She has her large share of medical problems and good food is major way to help balance her health. Did I mention she is GORGEOUS and my heart and soul?!

When she was about five years old, Lady C was diagnosed with mitral heart valve disease and an accompanying soft heart murmur (grade 3/6 diagnosed at Oregon State University, which included a 64-slice CT scan. They have an excellent canine cardiology program). She was about 4-5 pounds overweight at the time, which I attributed to mio Italiano spouse who loves through food (large amounts of it)! She immediately went on a diet, with measured food intake, and lost the extra weight. At her next two heart check-ups, she was downgraded to a 1/6 by the same cardiologist. Even though there is no scientific connection between MVD/murmur and weight loss, there was definitely a correlation with Lady C's heart condition. Fast forward to now, five years later, and she is still amazingly graded 2-3/6 with a soft murmur, with no prescribed heart medicine yet recommended.

Lady C also has other major medical issues, including PSOM (Primary Secretory Otitis Media diagnosed via MRI at UC Davis), facial nerve paralysis, and the worst one, Cushing's Disease (diagnosed via extensive testing at Oregon State University, Corvallis). She has more doctors than me, including an internist, cardiologist, dermatologist, ophthalmologist, neurologist, and general veterinarian.

She was diagnosed with Cushing's Disease (hyperadrenocorticism) in the summer of 2014. It started with elevated liver enzymes at a pre-dental blood screening, which lead to further investigation. She has the more common pituitary-type, which is a small tumor on the pituitary gland (near the brain and inoperable), which is the catalyst to an overproduction of cortisol via the adrenal glands. It is a very complex disease, and frustrating and difficult to treat at times. It is an autoimmune disease, which creates great susceptibility to infections. Untreated, it can lead to high blood pressure, stroke, diabetes, skin disease, organ failure and myriad other complications. Even with treatment, there are many complications. The pharmaceuticals are considered very strong and ongoing testing is required to monitor and adjust dosing.

When Lady was first diagnosed, I consulted with integrative veterinarian, Dr. Judy Morgan, to ascertain holistic treatment options. We tried a strict holistic routine for about a month, but the disease was progressing too quickly and she had to take the medication. Even with the medication, her immune system and metabolism were compromised and needed all possible help. I thought if humans with cancer and autoimmune disorders are helped with certain super foods, maybe such a diet could help Lady C. I wanted the best for her and wanted her to live as long and comfortable life as possible. So I used foods suggested by Dr. Morgan via consultation and later her book; plus adrenal supplements for adrenal gland health, milk thistle and Sam-e for liver health, and omega 3's and coconut oil for skin health. I also added to her daily diet: pumpkin and yogurt for digestive health, cranberries for urinary tract health, radishes and pears for cooling, blueberries for autoimmune health and my own creation, Super Food Stew!

Super Food Stew: I started making a major portion of Lady C's diet using all organic, healthy vegetables and a few fruits. I also added hormone free, grass feed meats such as chicken breast and beef. I more often use Alaskan white cod fish now. I cook the meat separately from the vegetables. For the vegetables, I chop them and then blanch them for about 10 minutes, starting with the carrots so they cook a little longer. I add any fruit right at the end, so they only boil about 2 minutes. Due to sugar content, I use limited fruit. After mixing the veggies/fruit with the meat, I separate into containers with 3-4 day portions. I freeze the extra portions and defrost a container in the fridge every 3 days or so. I make 2-4 weeks' worth of food at a time. (I do not feed the veggies raw since she appears to like the cooked ones better and with her, they digest better).

I vary the veggies and fruit, but use several kinds at once (all fresh, no canned): green beans, carrots, celery, squash, zucchini, kale, spinach, cranberries, Asian pears, apple and others. Sometimes there is a treat, like rinsed baby clams or wild salmon.

To make sure Lady C gets the daily recommended nutrients, I either add powdered vitamins or supplement one or two meals a day with The Honest Kitchen Preference and add the protein myself. It should be mentioned that the Cushing's has greatly affected Lady C's metabolism. In the past, she easily gained weight. Now I feed her 4-5 meals a day just to maintain her weight. So remember every dog is different and their needs can change over their lifetime or during a particular health issue. Always consult a veterinarian before making any changes!

Lady C has been eating 'good dog food' for a couple years now and I believe it has made a healthy difference. Me, not so much. I continue to indulge in sweets and processed foods at times. But I have learned a lot about nutrition from HER diet! I have NEVER given her table scraps in 10 years, but now think her table scraps would be better than mine!!

SNOODS FOR DOGS

Anyone who has a long-haired, long-eared dog knows that feeding raw or home cooked food can result in ears dragging through the moist food in the bowl. We've found our dogs happily chomping on their ears, trying to remove the last remains of dinner (a situation not dissimilar to men with beards and mustaches). After many episodes of washing and de-matting ears, we discovered there is a solution: SNOODS. Snoods are made to cover the head, holding the ears out of the way during meals. They can be knitted, crocheted, or sewn out of fanciful material. We like to purchase snoods with personality. We currently own snood lions, tigers, and panda, koala, and brown bears (Oh My!); apples, frogs, flowers, sheep, devils, mice, rabbits, giraffes, bumble bees, lady bugs, pigs, and leopards. All, of course, in brightly colored fun fabrics. Not only do these make great ear covers during meals, but they can also be transformed into a quick Halloween costume. We purchase our snoods from Day Dog Design on Etsy.com, but there are many places where they can be purchased.

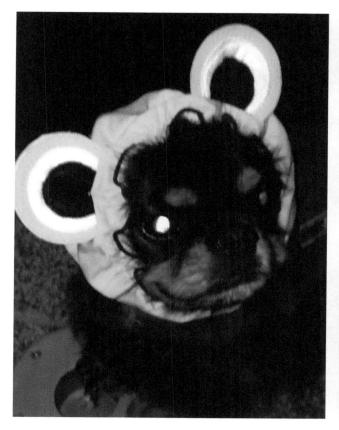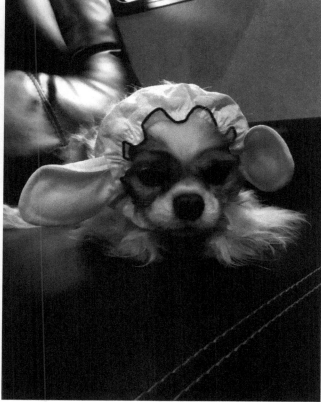

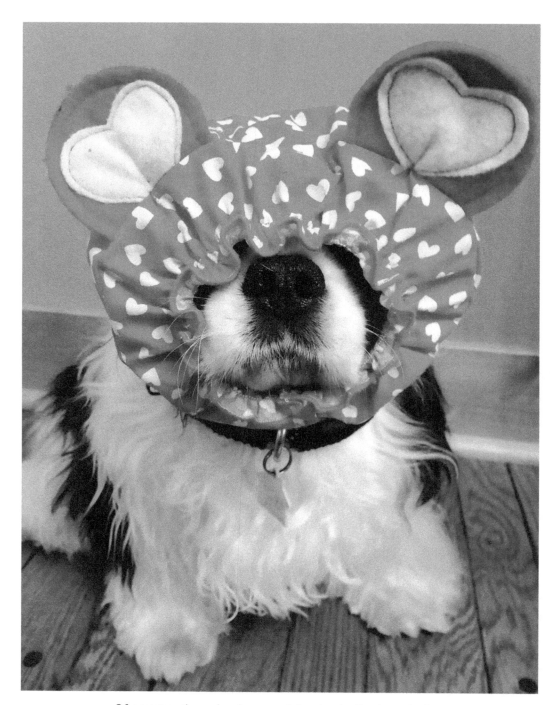

Of course, there is always a jokester in the bunch that
just can't figure out how to wear the snood properly...

HEAVENLY LEMON MERINGUE PIE FOR PEOPLE WITH A SWEET TOOTH

Submitted by Hue Grant

Ingredients:

1 recipe Sweet Pie Crust, recipe follows

1 recipe Italian Meringue, recipe follows

1 recipe Lemon Pie Filling, recipe follows

Directions

Sweet Pie Crust:

1 1/4 cups all-purpose flour

1 tablespoon sugar

1/4 teaspoon salt

6 tablespoons cold, unsalted butter, cut into pieces

2 tablespoons cold vegetable shortening

3 to 4 tablespoons ice water, or as needed

Sift the flour, sugar, and salt into a large bowl. With your fingers, work the butter and shortening into the dry ingredients until the mixture resembles coarse crumbs. Add 3 tablespoons of the ice water and work with your fingers just until the dough comes together, adding more water as needed, 1 teaspoon at a time, to make a smooth dough, being careful not to overwork the dough. Form the dough into a disk shape, wrap tightly in plastic wrap, and refrigerate for at least 30 minutes before using.

Yield: enough dough for 1 (9 or 10-inch) crust

Remove the dough from the refrigerator; on a lightly floured surface, roll out to a 12-inch circle. Transfer the dough to a 9-inch pie pan, pressing gently to fit, trim the edge to within 1/2-inch of the pan, turn under, and crimp decoratively. Refrigerate for 30 minutes to 1 hour.

Preheat the oven to 375 degrees F.

Line the pie shell with parchment paper and fill with pie weights, dry beans, or rice. Bake until crust is set, about 12 minutes. Remove the parchment paper and weights and bake until lightly colored, 8 to 10 minutes. Cool on a wire rack before filling.

Filling:

　　　　1 1/4 cups granulated sugar

　　　　5 tablespoons cornstarch

　　　　1 cup milk

　　　　1/2 cup cold water

　　　　1/8 teaspoon salt

　　　　6 large egg yolks

　　　　2/3 cup fresh lemon juice

　　　　2 tablespoons finely grated lemon zest

　　　　1 1/2 tablespoons limoncello

　　　　2 tablespoons cold unsalted butter, cut into pieces

Combine the granulated sugar, cornstarch, milk, water, and pinch of the salt in a large, non-reactive saucepan, whisk to combine, and bring to a simmer over medium heat, whisking occasionally. As the mixture reaches a simmer and begins to thicken and turn clear, 4 to 5 minutes, whisk in the egg yolks, 2 at a time. Slowly add the lemon juice, whisking constantly, and add the zest and limoncello. Add the butter, 1 piece at a time, and whisking constantly, return to a simmer. Remove from the heat and pour immediately into the prepared pie crust.

Meringue:

1 cup superfine sugar

1/3 cup water

6 egg whites, at room temperature

1/4 teaspoon cream of tartar

In a small pot over low heat, combine sugar and water. Swirl the pot over the burner to dissolve the sugar completely. Do not stir. Increase the heat and boil to soft-ball stage (235 to 240 degrees). Use a candy thermometer for accuracy. Wash down the inside wall of the pot with a wet pastry brush. This will help prevent sugar crystals from forming around the sides, falling in and causing a chain reaction.

Prepare your meringue:

In the bowl of an electric mixer, whip the eggs whites on low speed until foamy. Add the cream of tartar, increase the speed to medium, and beat until soft peaks form. With the mixer running, pour the hot sugar syrup in a thin stream over fluffed egg whites. Beat until the egg whites are stiff and glossy.

Spread the meringue evenly over the hot pie filling using a rubber spatula, smoothing out to the pastry edges. Make decorative peaks in the meringue using a dull knife or the back of a spoon.) To quickly cook the meringue, preheat the broiler with the rack in the highest position. Place the pie under the broiler and cook until the meringue is set and golden brown, 1 to 2 minutes, watching carefully to avoid burning. (Alternatively, the meringue can be cooked in a preheated 325 degree F oven until set and golden brown, 14 to 16 minutes.) Transfer the pie to a wire rack to cool completely before serving.

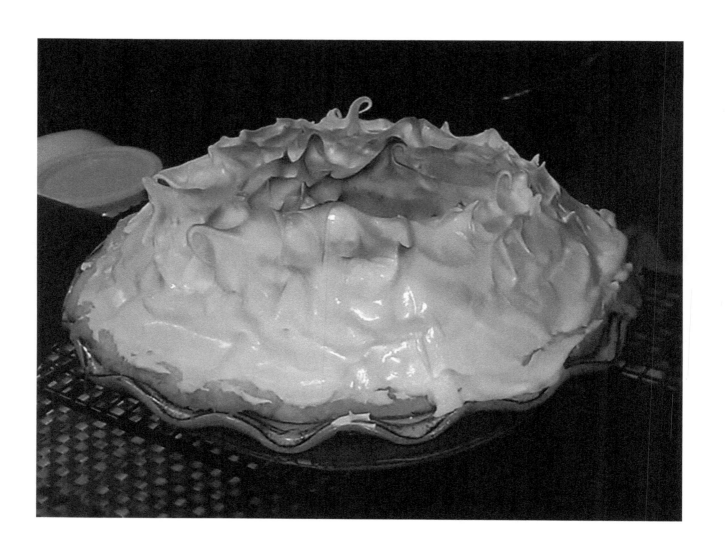

NEIGHBORS

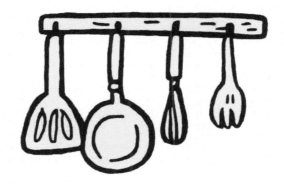

Submitted by Carol Oliver

My story, on a more serious note, involves a neighbor, Mrs J, and her Bichon Frise, Brie. (names changed). This occurred over a period of a couple years.

One day we noticed Brie scratching and biting at himself while out on the a.m. dog walk. His skin looked raw. Me: *What's wrong with Brie?*

Mrs J.: *Allergies.*

Me: *Maybe to the dog food? What do you feed?* (can't recall the response).

Weeks later...

Mrs J.: *Brie is much better. He had a shot of "something" and has these antibiotics. I think he's all better now.*

Me: Thinking *Don't be so sure.* Responded with *Great!*

Months later....

Mrs J.: *Well, Brie was scratching like crazy again, I had to bring him back to the vet. She gave him another shot. He was due for other shots anyway. And now we have antibiotics to give and Prednisone.*

Me: *Perhaps you shouldn't give shots anymore. You especially should not give several on the same day.* Reminded her that Prednisone and other medications can be lifesavers in emergencies, but are also Band-Aids that mask the symptoms without treating the underlying cause. Cautiously readdressed *What do you feed him?*

More Months later, Brie is wearing a cone. The cone is worn out on the lower side.

Me: *What happened to Brie? What's with the cone? Surgery?*

Mrs J.: *Oh, this is the only way we can keep him from biting and scratching. He's making his skin raw and going crazy.*

Me: *Have you considered changing the diet? Many health issues are due to diet alone. Would you like me to help with food?*

Mrs J.: *Oh no, my vet has him on a special diet* < brand omitted>. *And we increased the Prednisone.*

We did not see Brie for quite some time after. When we did, he looked pathetic.

Brie wears the hard plastic cone 24/7 now, has severe hair loss, raw red skin, distended belly, severe panting, his head is lowered, eyes looking up...pleading. Clearly depressed.

Me: *Poor boy, he looks absolutely miserable, plus he has Cushing's Disease.*

Mrs J.: *He doesn't have Cushing's. We had him tested for that years ago.*

Me: *Well he does now; it's called iatrogenic, meaning the disease is caused by other medical treatment, namely the Prednisone.* Discussed in greater detail. (Writer is an advanced practice nurse.)

Mrs J.: *We can't increase the Prednisone any more, he's on a maximum dose now. He's constantly drinking and peeing every minute, everywhere. He's panting constantly. I just don't know what to do. Is the only other alternative at this point to put him to sleep?*

Imagine this image - The dog really did look like he was pleading with us to please end his life. It just broke my heart. <all teary eyed now>

Me: <pleading> *Please, can we try my homemade dog food?*

Mrs J.: *I don't have the time to make that.*

Me: *So instead you must make the time for veterinary visits, plus take time off from work?*

Mrs J.: *Well, I can't afford it.*

Me: *But you can afford the costly veterinary visits, treatment, medications, and the costly commercial prescription food?* (and this is a very expensive area) *PLUS and MOST importantly, this is not to mention how the poor dog is suffering! What have you got to lose at this point? Please, if you pay for half the ingredients, I will make the food for you, just promise you won't feed that other garbage.*

I finally convinced Mrs J to try my food. After all, what did she have to lose? At first the dog was a little puzzled by his strange new food, but thought it was yummy. After a couple days, he couldn't wait for his meals. Within 3 weeks, Mrs J admitted in a surprised tone: *You know, I think he might be scratching less.* Me: *Wonderful!*

I invited her over to assist in the next batch of food preparation. She was a bit overwhelmed at first, but I reminded her that it was less time and effort than vet visits and less costly too, plus the dog liked it and was improving; a win, win, win situation. Plus, once Mrs J learned the process, I knew she would create her own preparation plan and learn how to save time. Mrs. J was now a believer and thrilled beyond belief.

After 3 months the dog's condition had significantly improved. The prednisone was tapered, the skin began to improve, his Cushing's signs and symptoms were resolving, his panting all but disappeared, the excessive drinking and peeing had resolved. After 3-6 months' time, Brie was growing new hair, and his distended abdomen was beginning to show signs of improvement. Most importantly, his expression changed from sad and depressed to the happy boy he once used to be. He regained that bounce in his step.

Her (conventional) vet's comments: *I can't believe it. Hmmm, maybe it was the food.*

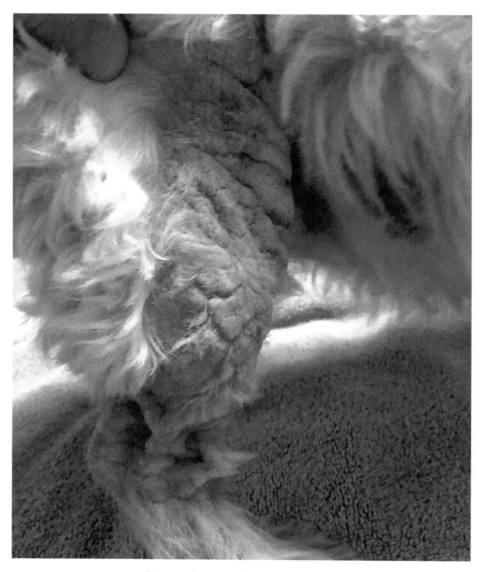

The misery of food allergy.

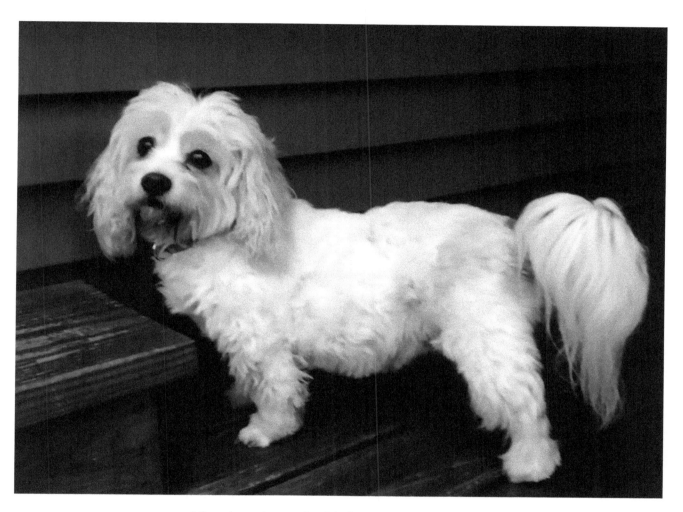

Allergies cleared with home cooked food!

RABBIT STEW FOR ALLERGY DOGS

Submitted by Judy Morgan DVM

6 pounds cut up rabbit pieces (I get them with bone; you can buy de-boned, but it's expensive)

2 pounds rabbit organs

1 turnip

3 carrots

1 cup chopped kale

1/2 cup parsley

1 cup cranberries

Grind or finely chop the veggies, fruits, and organs. Mix with the meat in a crock pot and cover with 4 cups water. Cook on high for 4 hours, allow to remain on warm setting for one hour. (I actually let it just sit over-night.) De-bone the rabbit chunks, cool, and serve. A calcium/mineral supplement, a few drops Vitamin D3, and a probiotic should be added at the time of feeding.

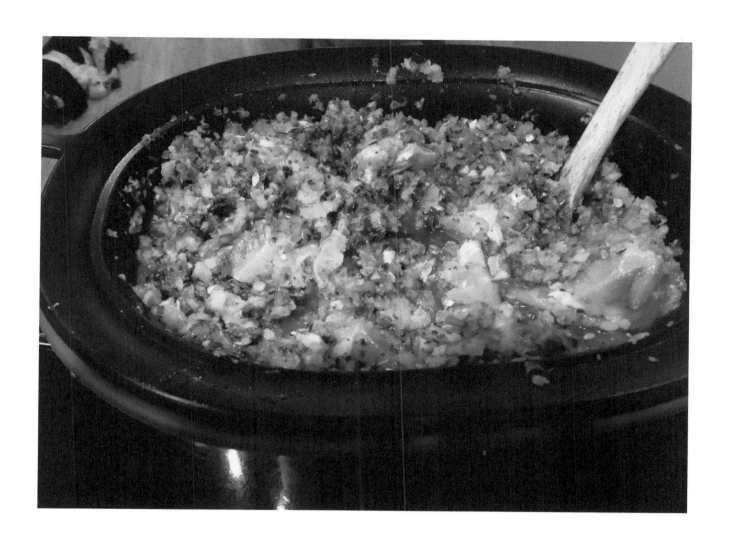

WHITE CHOCOLATE CHIP SNICKERDOODLE COOKIES FOR YOUR NEIGHBOR

(No nuts, just in case your neighbor has allergies. But seriously, you might not want to share.)

Submitted by Kirstyn Grant

1 ½ cups granulated sugar

½ cup softened butter

½ cup vegetable shortening

2 eggs

2 ¾ cups all purpose flour

2 teaspoons cream of tartar

1 teaspoon baking soda

¼ teaspoon table salt

¾ cup white chocolate chips

¼ cup sugar and 2 teaspoons cinnamon for topping

Directions:

Cream sugar, butter, and shortening together. Add in eggs and mix well.

In a separate bowl, sift together flour, cream of tartar, baking soda, and salt.

Combine wet ingredients into the dry and mix well. Stir in the white chocolate chips. Place the dough in the freezer to chill for 30 minutes.

Preheat your oven to 350 degrees. In a small bowl combine the sugar and cinnamon for the topping. Roll cookie dough into 1 inch balls, roll the balls in the sugar and cinnamon mixture. Place the balls of cookie dough on an ungreased baking sheet. Bake 14 to 16 minutes until the edges just start to brown. Centers should still be a little gooey. Remove and allow to cool on the

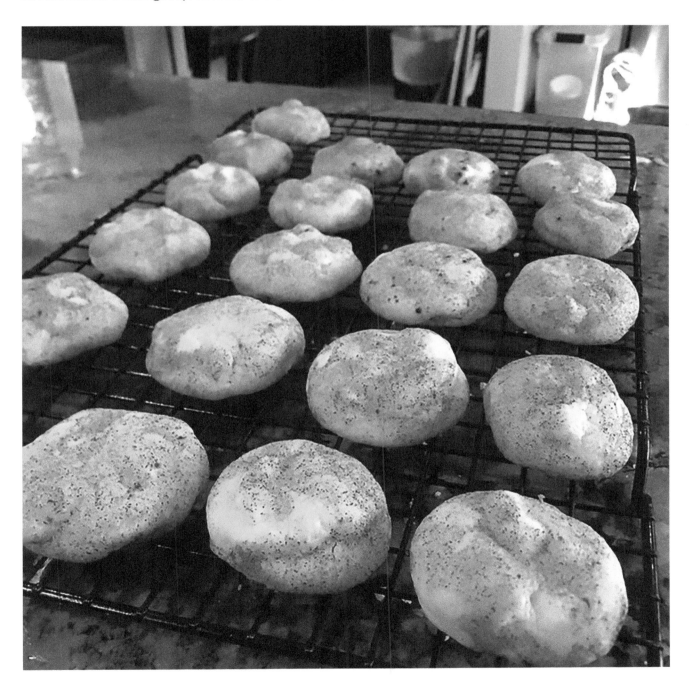

ROOM SERVICE

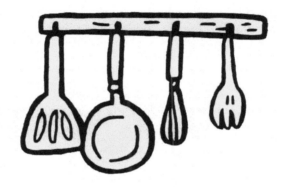

Submitted by Faith Jones

In 1994, cooking for your dog was not in vogue. Most of my friends and relatives thought I was a little off my rocker. But my 14 year old Cocker Spaniel had congestive heart failure and she required a low salt diet. I did not like the ingredients in the prescription food sold by my veterinarian. When I told him that, he gave me a copy of the Hill's Science Diet cookbook, which does not exist anymore.

I started making meals for my dog and things were going well, but we needed to travel five hundred miles to a large family reunion at a hotel in West Virginia. I figured if I could transport and store the meals safely, Nugget could accompany us and would be just fine during the trip. Nugget's meals were frozen individually and transported in our cooler. When I called to schedule our reservations at the hotel, I specified I needed a room with a refrigerator. However, upon check-in, we are told the refrigerator we reserved with our rooms was not available! I didn't know what to do with all the frozen meals in our cooler.

I stared at the hotel clerk while trying to think of a way around this dilemma. Normally I am an honest person, but for my dogs, I'll do what is needed! I told the clerk that I had to have a refrigerator as "I" was on a special diet. The manager was called and he told me that I could keep my food in the restaurant freezer.

The next day, I went to the kitchen for "my" food. They looked everywhere and could not find the large, marked package! The chef came out, apologized, and offered to cook whatever I needed. With a deep breath, I said I needed unsalted chicken breast, carrots and boiled rice! They did not have unsalted chicken or plain rice. Hmm, I had to think quickly!

I asked for unsalted broiled hamburger, peas, carrots and 2 baked potatoes. Room Service! The chef surely thought I was slightly disturbed; he could not understand why I wanted the same food every day. And this was delivered for 4 days! The last day, my husband told the chef the real story and we all had a good laugh together.

Lesson learned - if there is no refrigerator, keep food in your cooler and add ice, as needed. God bless little Nugget, who traveled with her crazy family until she left us at almost 17 years of age.

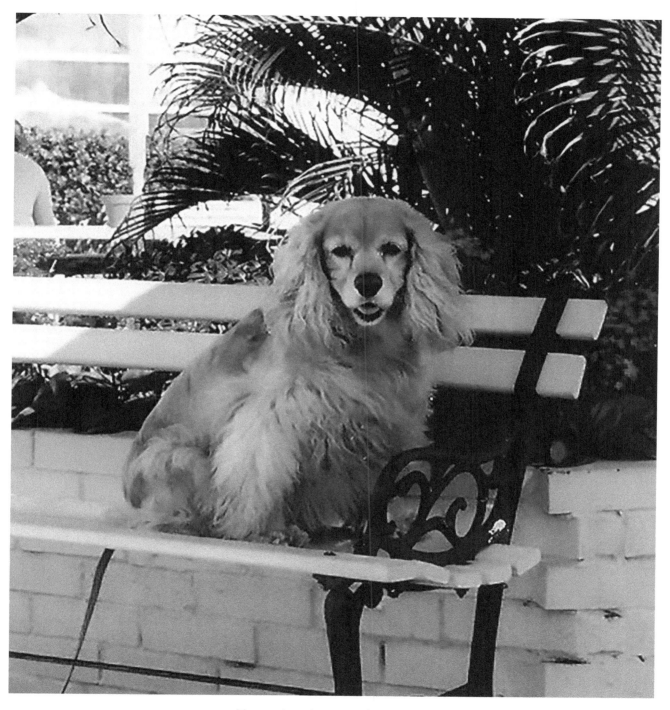

Nugget only gets the best!

HEART HEALTHY MEAL FOR DOGS

Submitted by Judy Morgan

2 pounds 93 to 96% lean ground beef

4 ounces beef heart with fat trimmed

2 ounces beef liver

1 cup chopped kale

1 cup chopped spinach

½ cup parsley chopped

½ cup grated carrots

4 ounces Shiitake mushrooms chopped

½ cup canned organic pumpkin

½ cup organic blueberries

2 eggs with shells (grind shells)

4 tsp cod liver oil

4 mussels minced

4 ounces wheat germ

Mix all ingredients together and pour into a loaf pan. Bake at 350 for about 45 minutes. Do not overcook. Contains about 580 calories per cup. Dogs should eat 20 to 30 calories per pound of body weight daily, depending on activity level. One cup per day will feed a 20 pound active dog or a 30 pound lazy dog (approximately).

HOW TO ORDER ROOM SERVICE

Decide on a wonderful vacation destination.

Book the best hotel you can find.

Inform your spouse the reservations are confirmed.

Upon arrival, ask the desk clerk the hours room service is available and which number to dial on the phone to get room service.

Approximately 45 minutes before your preferred meal time, call and request the nicest steak on the menu, with an appropriate bottle of wine.

Sit back and relax.

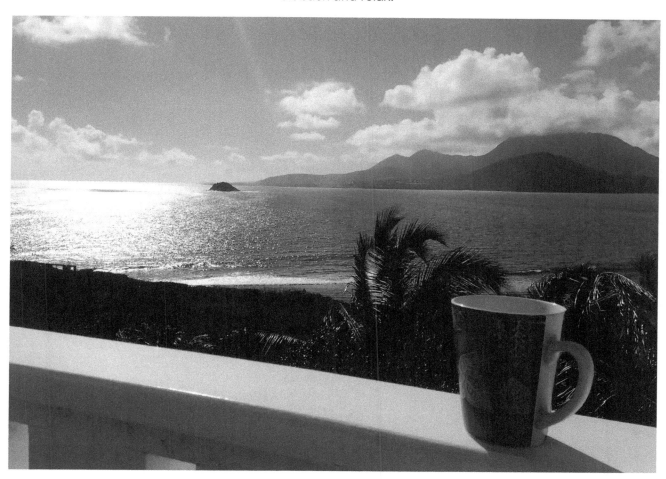

COOKING ON THE SABBATH

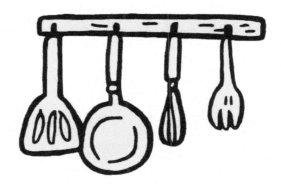

Submitted by Liz Vernon's Soldier, Lexi, Billy, and Rooney

Billy, Soldier, Lexi, and guest-- Rooney the Golden Doodle-- here. We have a witness to Mom's dimwitted-ness! Rooney is amazed. We are used to this; in fact we think maybe we should probably increase our term of "somewhat dimwitted" to something a little stronger. Mom mixed up more puppy loaves. Cuz Mom does not like to cook, although she sure likes to eat, she makes huge batches to freeze at a time. Everything was actually going according to plan, and Mom cooked the first three big loaves and a couple mini loaves in the first batch. Mom said all four of us were under her feet all the time, whatever that means; we just were sticking close to meatloaf production.

Mom got the second batch ready to go and her oven had a strange new code on it. She couldn't get any controls to work. Mom hates this oven; it was a replacement to the one that blew up. Yes, blew up. Mom's friends and former neighbors were visiting and the oven started flaming and sparking and Billy says it was spectacular. Her friends were laughing; they said Mom would do ANYTHING to get out of cooking. Mom hadn't realized that the big lightning strike a couple weeks before had blown out the oven, cuz she usually uses the toaster broiler. That's what she says happened. Really.

Mom did something she would normally never do; she sent Dad out to get a new oven, since she had guests. Mom is always accidentally hitting a button that puts it in a different mode. Even just trying to clean it, she hits buttons. She keeps the manual handy, cuz it happens so much. And now the oven wouldn't work. This was something new, though. Mom looked it up; it took her a long time to find what "SAB" meant.

To Mom's great surprise, we have an oven that will observe Sabbath. While Mom has great respect for Sabbath, she wasn't trying to observe it, she was just trying to make our puppy loaves...but ya know, some-thing always seems to happen. And of course, because Mom marches to a different drum, she managed to create her own special Sabbath time, not the official date of Sabbath. Yep, Mom locked our oven in Sab-bath mode. Mom was expecting to find a way to clear the lock-out; instead she read that no controls would function for 11.5 hours. Mom had been working on a schedule. Mom always has schedules and plans; we don't know why, because 99% of them do not work out the way she planned. Mom likes to pretend she has some control over life. Mom told Dad what happened. Dad looked at Mom incredulously, like he always does when she has another one of her fiascoes. Neither she nor we know why, after thirty years, he is still surprised by this kind of thing. He asked if she had tried flipping the electrical fuse for the oven. Mom never thought of that; great idea. Dad went and flipped the fuse and left it off for five minutes. Still in Sabbath. Then he left it off for half-hour; oven still in Sabbath. Mom announced we had a strictly orthodox oven. Mom says she could understand being locked out of an oven if there was chocolate in it, since she is a chocoholic, but she doesn't understand why someone observing Sabbath has to go so far as having their oven locked, since they wouldn't be cooking anyway. She is confused, but as you know, that's nothing new, either.

Dad told Mom not to do this one again. Mom glared at Dad because she doesn't usually repeat her fias-coes; she goes on to different ones, but in this event she has no idea how she got into Sabbath mode and she had already told Dad that, cuz every time she has a new "episode", he always asks "How did THIS happen?". Dad likes to pretend he has some control over Mom. We don't know who is dreaming more, Mom with her plans or Dad with that illusion.

So, Mom had to fit the huge industrial mixing bowl full of meatloaf guts in the refrigerator and the loaves she had had ready to go in. She had the nerve to ask her neighbor, who is already letting her use her freezer for frozen beef heart and livers, if she could borrow space in her fridge overnight. Lucky for her, our neighbor hates to cook as much as Mom and is happy Mom is giving her a puppy loaf for her Cocker Spaniel or a human loaf for her every time she is in mass production mode of those.

Today, our oven has declared we are done observing Sabbath. Rooney the doodle is very happy cuz it's been a couple years since Mom and Dad had a big dog that could just reach over on the counter and grab something. Mom forgot about scooting everything two feet back. Rooney got a loaf, and since she is so easy going, we all got to share it. All Mom did was go to the mailbox and came back to us licking the last remains. Mom says we just ate three days worth of food. She's crazy; it was JUST a little snack. It's been a very good day! We all hope you have as good a day!

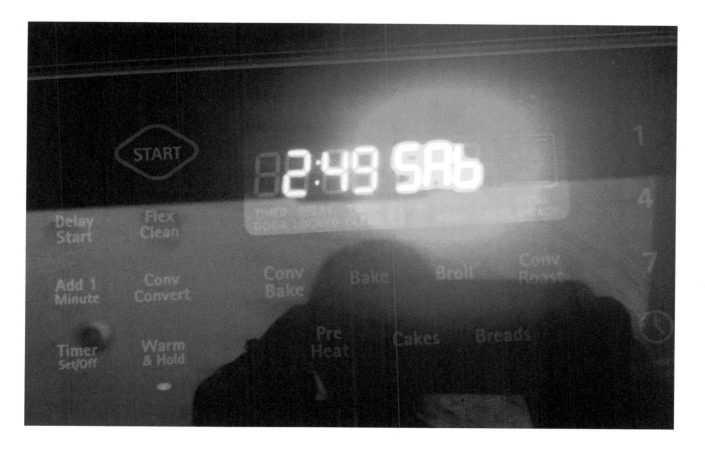

MAKING RESERVATIONS FOR DINNER WHEN THE STOVE IS STUCK ON SABBATH

1. **Call as far ahead of time as possible.** In many cases, you'll be able to make a dinner reservation early in the same day. Of course, if you have just spent all day cooking for the dogs, you may be making this call at the last minute.

2. **Schedule an early or late dinner if availability is limited.** Eating at 5 pm or 10 pm doesn't really matter, as long as someone else is doing the cooking.

3. **Be as courteous as possible when booking a reservation.** Remember that your attitude on the phone will go a long way. Be confident but polite; avoid giving the impression that you feel entitled to a reservation (which, of course, you are, because you just spent all day cooking for dogs!) If the host responds that the restaurant has no availability, explain your situation and ask politely if there is any way to squeeze you in. As a last resort, cry.

4. **Once you've conned your way into a reservation, call ahead if you are running late.** (Which of course you will be by the time you finish washing green slime off your cabinets and cleaning the blender, grinder, mallet, utensils, pots, and pans.)

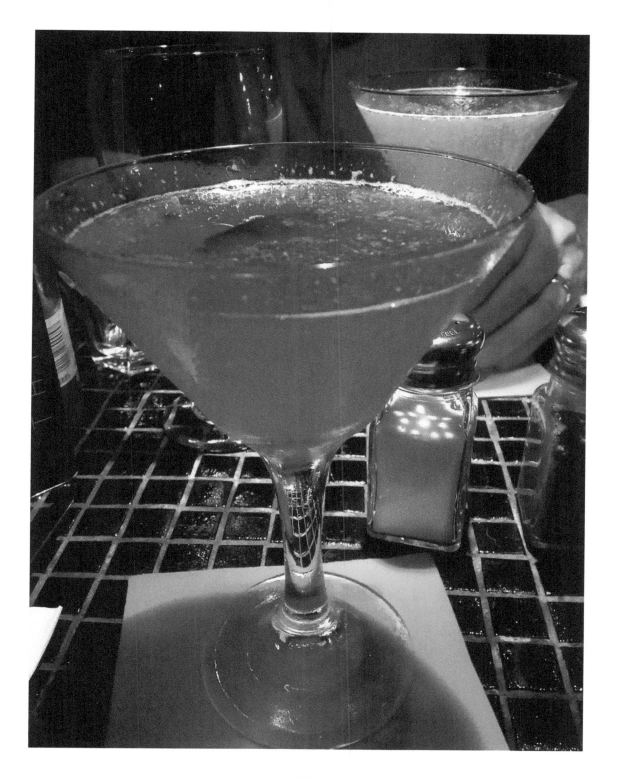

FEAST OF THE SEVEN FISHES

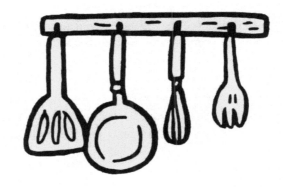

Submitted by Hue Grant

Life with Judy is always interesting, to say the least. My mantra, over time, has become "expect the unexpected". To this end, I was curious when I rolled over at 3:00 a.m. on a December Sunday to find her laptop glowing while she feverishly typed away...

Curious, but still sleepy, I rolled back over, snuggled with the spaniels and drifted back into dreamland. I awoke at a more reasonable time, to find her and the spaniels anxiously waiting to share something. Judy said she wanted to create a special recipe for the spaniels' Christmas Eve dinner. Rubbing my eyes, I thought why not? She's probably thinking about some tweak to her puploaf or maybe a nice beef stew; so I asked what she had in mind. Famous last words...

She grinned and exclaimed that we were going to make a feast of seven fishes! Judy then shared that, during her nocturnal research, she had been messaging back and forth with Facebook friends to glean information about the traditional meal of seven fishes and had actually even gotten feedback from friends in Italy. She also said that she was being a little bit secretive because she wanted this to be a surprise Christmas post. Most of her friends thought she was asking about the feast so that we could cook a meal for ourselves, not the dogs.

Knowing that we were going to run headlong into this project, I suggested that a trip to the grocery store was in order to see what products might be available and that she should also think about how this might all be prepared. Of course, she was way ahead of me and offered that she wanted it to be a stew that included things like mushrooms, butternut squash, and kale.

So, with only five days until Christmas, I headed to grocery store to fight the crowds and explore the fish counter. Now, being from Texas, I usually spend most of my time looking at the meat case and drooling over the ribeye steaks, prime rib roasts and thick pork chops. I was surprised to see so many options in the fish case. There was squid and octopus and various white fish, salmon and tuna, and all kinds of shellfish. There was also a sign that advertised a sale on seafood to create your own feast of seven fishes. Maybe this would work!

Upon arriving back home, I shared the fruits of my research and Judy got busy designing our recipe. I, on the other hand, starting looking up various fish stew recipes to determine how difficult it might be to work with seafood that I had never eaten, much less prepared. By mid-afternoon, as always happens, we both got consumed with other projects, horses, spaniels, and life, so it was determined that we would prepare the spaniels' feast on Tuesday, our day off.

Fast-forward to Tuesday morning, two days before Christmas. Off we went to the store in search of our feast ingredients. Staring down through the glass display case, the first thing I noticed was an octopus staring back at me. I bravely pointed to it and asked the clerk to pick it up. This was the clerk that usually helped me, so she asked her usual question. "Is this for you or is it for the dogs?" She didn't even flinch when I explained that we were creating a feast of seven fishes for the spaniels. Next I selected a piece of swordfish, then some clams, several smelt, flounder and squid. We had already decided that we would add canned sardines, so with that rounding out our seven fishes, we gathered the produce we needed and headed for the checkout. Now, if you have ever ventured to the grocery store two days before Christmas, you know that only crazed maniacs, resorting to the last minute rush, are present. You also know that we waited in one of a dozen lines that stretched back to the rear of the store in order to finalize our purchase and head home.

Arriving home, we unpacked our bags and gathered pans and utensils. But wait! We couldn't just start slicing and dicing; we had to stage a display of ingredients for the obligatory photo shoot so that the recipe post for Facebook would be complete.

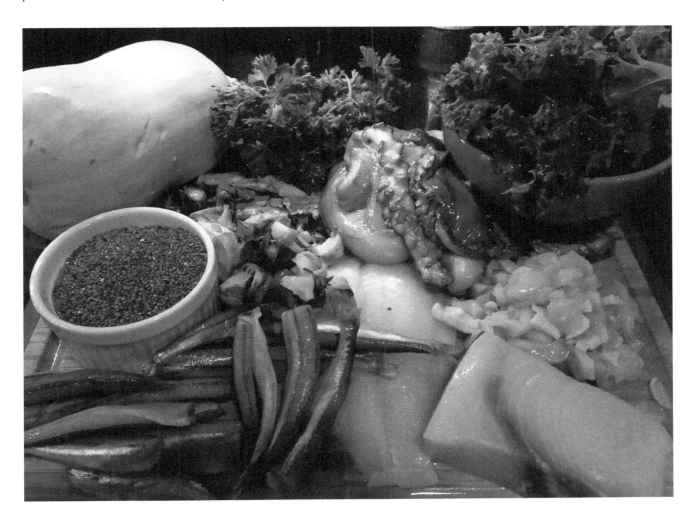

Here again, I'm a beef person; I've never thought twice about handling any part of the cow. I've even prepared mountain oysters without flinching. But, handling the octopus was a new and slimy treat. The closest I had been to an octopus, previously, was the movie theatre watching *Twenty Thousand Leagues Under the Sea*.

In any event, I grabbed Mister Octopus and held him up for a photo. When stretched out on the counter top, he measured almost three feet long! I dipped him in the pot of boiling water and watched him shrivel, just as the Internet recipe page had hastily taught me the day before.

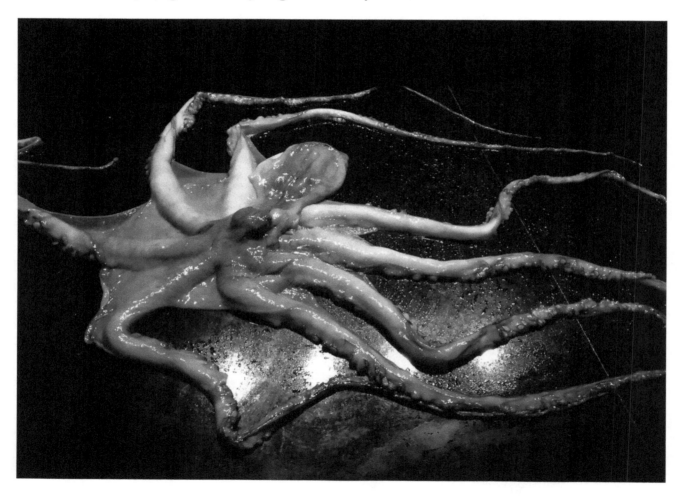

With all the clamoring around the kitchen, the Spaniels, as they always intuitively know, started milling around to soak up the smells. They made attempts to trip us up, with the hope that a tasty morsel might drop or spill. Without missing a beat, we all waltzed around the kitchen, finally managing to get all the ingredients into the stewpot.

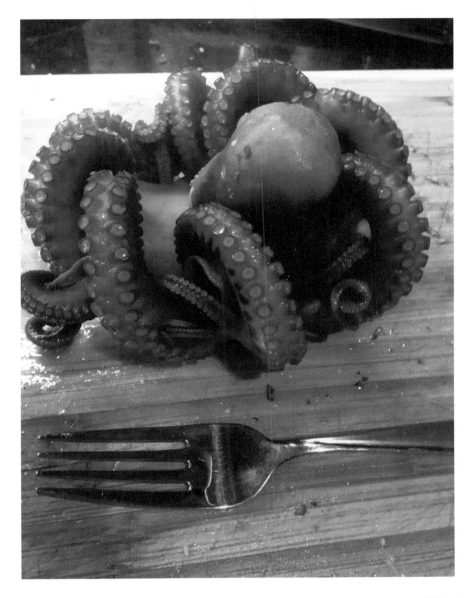

Fortunately, a fish stew doesn't need a lot of time on the stove, so by 5 p.m. we were filling bowls and trying to convince spaniels that it was in their best interest to let everything cool a bit. During this cool-down period, Judy looked over at me and asked what I was serving for the human dinner. Without missing a beat, I replied, martinis and cheese!

So while Spaniels made happy slurping sounds I shook the martinis, sliced cheese, put out an assortment of crackers, and we all feasted to Christmas music playing in the background.

FIDO'S FEAST OF THE SEVEN FISHES

Submitted by Judy Morgan

1 pound Swordfish cut up

1 pound Clams chopped

1 small Octopus – see preparation below

½ pound Smelt cut up

½ pound Squid cut up

½ pound Flounder cut up

3 cans (3.75 ounce each) Sardines in water

4 ounces Shiitake Mushrooms chopped

8 ounces Kale chopped

1 bunch Parsley chopped

1 medium Butternut squash peeled and cubed

1 cup Red quinoa

Dip octopus in boiling water 3 times, allowing tentacles to shrink. Then put in boiling water for 20 minutes. Turn off heat and allow to sit in water for an additional 20 minutes. Remove and cool. Cut off head and discard. Cut tentacles into small pieces.

Cut up all other ingredients and place in stew pot. Simmer together for 45 to 60 minutes. Cool and mix in octopus pieces. Serve as a special meal.

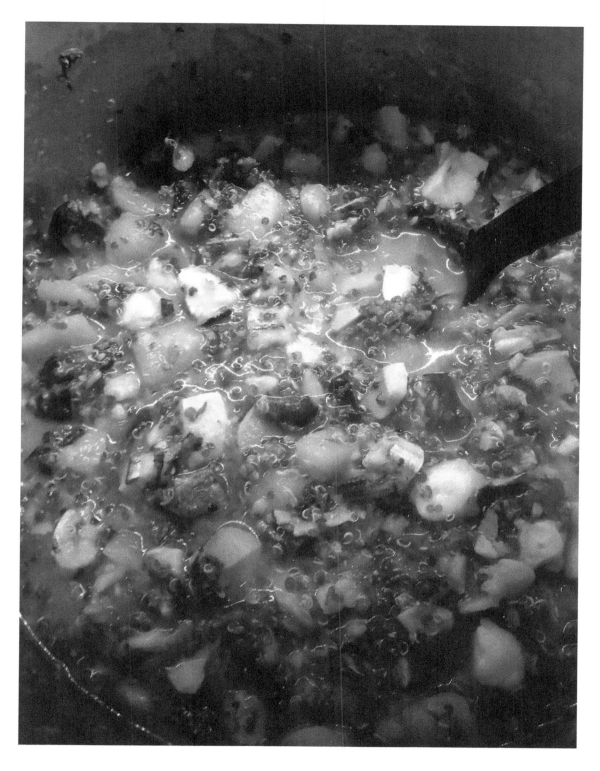

CHRISTMAS MARTINIS AND CHEESE

1. Everyday gin is Burnetts (or whatever is available) but, for the holidays, splurge and break out the Bombay Sapphire.

2. Fill metal shaker halfway with ice cubes, then add as much gin as the shaker will hold. This is one time size really does matter.

3. Shake said shaker vigorously for one minute or until ice crystals form on the metal surface. As Bond always says, martinis should be shaken, not stirred.

4. Pour into clean martini glasses. Festive Christmas glasses are preferred for the holidays.

5. Slice a selection of cheeses, hoping that there are more than Kraft singles in the refrigerator. If Kraft singles are the only cheese available, make the slices more appealing by rolling into tubes or cutting into festive holiday shapes. Also, make sure you slice an ample amount because the task becomes more difficult and dangerous after a couple of martinis.

6. Place crackers on a tray. Bonus points if they aren't stale.

7. Dream up a sappy toast and serve.

8. Repeat steps 2 thru 4 as often as necessary.

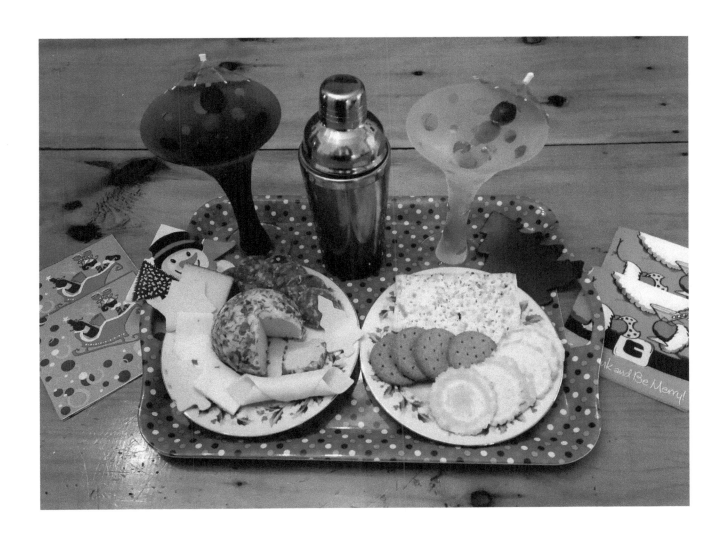

READY, SET, COOK!

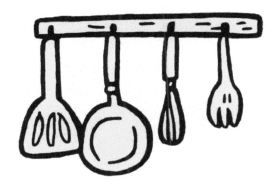

Now that we've given you all these great recipes and ideas, you have no excuse to forego making food for your dogs. If all the wonderful pet parents in these stories have managed to keep their homes from burning down and their spouses from leaving home, we think that's enough reason to get started. Your dogs will be healthier and happier when you do. Start with something simple and work your way up to gourmet meals.

If you find yourself getting overwhelmed, we've given you the tools to order take-out or room service or to make a quick meal of hot dogs, popcorn, martinis, and crackers. If things don't go well and you find yourself in the middle of a disaster, be sure to get good photos and send them to us. Not only will we be sure to share them on social media, but you might just get your own chapter in our next project.

Happy cooking!

Sincerely,

Judy and Hue